THE
EXTRAORDINARY
ORDINARY
YOU

A MANUAL FOR SELF DISCOVERY

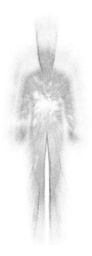

Danielle L. Brooks

The Extraordinary Ordinary You
A Manual for Self Discovery
By Danielle L. Brooks

Library of Congress Control Number: 2023901453
Ebook ISBN: 979-8-9872920-0-6
Hardback ISBN: 979-8-9872920-1-3
Paperback ISBN: 979-8-9872920-2-0

Published by:
Good Decisions, Inc
Jackson WY
425 445-9065
www.daniellebrooks.com

Printed in the United States of America

TABLE OF CONTENTS

INTRODUCTION

The information in this book includes my personal experiences and those of the clients who I help guide, but the information is much bigger than that. It marks the dawning of a new day. I've worked with hundreds of individuals at various stages of awakening and I can assure you, there is a wave coming, a wave of consciousness so profound and so life changing no one will be able to stop it. And who would want to? This wave represents the crashing down of what is not real and illuminates, like a glorious phosphorescent wave, the truth.

Humanity has been creating from a false template of separation for eons. This has been necessary in order for Oneness to spring forth into the physical as a subject and an object, as you and me. Physicality needs polarity. We need north and south, up and down, left and right. We need space and time to exist in this physical realm; otherwise, how would the blood in your veins move from your heart to your head? This is polarity. But somewhere along the way polarity got distorted and we forgot the truth of our being. We forgot that we all exist in a field of

Oneness that connects all things and all beings. Oneness in its forgetfulness became separation and opposition. But now we are remembering. Individuals all over the world are waking up to themselves as connected to a greater expansive beingness. I have the great honor of seeing it every day, and it is beautiful beyond description. The wave is coming!

If you choose to hop on that wave you will have the ride of your life. If you decide to stay stagnant things will be difficult. Have you noticed that waves only pummel the things that don't move? This book is a manual designed to help you move. It is designed to aid you in letting go of what you are not so you can float to the surface and ride the wave.

It will remind you not to take awakening so seriously. The more you are playful at heart, the greater the ride will be. When you live with the open heart of a child you are able to receive information that can trigger your memory of who and what you are. This is wonderful! When you know who you are, everything of non-importance drops away and the next thing you know you are hanging ten on a surfboard acting like a puppy wagging its tail at seeing yourself come home.

The information you receive from this book will tickle you. You are ready for it. Information is often received via an insight, realization, or inner knowing. Stay open to it. Imagine as you turn the pages that you are two years old again and you are learning about the world for the very first time. Participate in the great unknowing by forgetting everything you think you know and be in a state of wonder; take pleasure in the possibilities, let your imagination run wild. The fact that you found your way to this book is an indication that your surfboard is in hand and you are looking out at the ocean with excitement. You see the wave coming and can't wait! In fact, you're already riding it.

Welcome home to the great expanse!

You Are a Powerful Creator

Everything in this book is based on the primary foundation that you, my dearest, are a powerful creator. Who you are in your innermost being—whether it is called source energy, oneness, pure consciousness individuated, God particle, or true self— matters not. You are an extraordinary being. And you create in this realm via choice, self awareness, and vibrational alignment. A choice is the same thing as an intention, so for clarity's sake we will use the word choice throughout this text. For instance, when you intend to go to the bathroom, you choose to. When you intend to quit your job, make a sandwich, or give your sweetheart a kiss, you choose to.

Many of us create unconsciously; we go through our days unaware of the thoughts bouncing around in our minds and go through the hours in the day habitually, sometimes never even remembering the drive home. We just aren't present.

And some of us create consciously. Conscious creators know themselves to be connected to something greater. They know themselves as unlimited beings that are visiting a created reality. They have mastered the ability to choose which thoughts and feelings they would like to align to in order to create their reality. They know how to come vibrationally into alignment with their desires, and are free to create anything without judgment. They choose what they would like to experience and boom! They're in the Virtual Reality (VR) room of their own design. They know there is no good or bad or right or wrong; there is only experience for the sake of experience. In many ways the VR room helps you understand and answer the questions: Who am I? What can I become?

You gain wisdom with every experience. It's like taking a trip to the amusement park where you are free to hop on any ride you desire, and so is everyone else. There is no judgment, no fear, no guilt, no shame, no should or shouldn't, no rights or wrongs, no need to or have to.

None of that.

Only unlimited freedom, choice, experience, and expression.

Sounds pretty cool, right? This is called undistorted creation. Undistorted creation is creation that occurs in full awareness.

My friend and mentor Lauri Ivers has walked with me on my journey for over three years. She is the clearest channel and intuitive guide I have ever met. She has challenged me to develop my own intuitive abilities, to become a clear and undistorted channel of truth, and has been the teacher that showed up for me when I, as a student, was ready. The thing that makes her such an excellent guide is her willingness to be on the journey with me. She allows me to challenge her; she encourages it. Together we have grown beyond our imaginations. For every question I had, she dipped into the quantum field and brought through with clarity and precision the truth and showed me how to do it. I know it is truth because of how my body responds. The body recognizes the truth when it lands because it lands as a knowing. Lauri has no interest in being significant or special. She knows that which lives within her lies within all beings. Her sole desire is to wake up others to their own divinity, sovereignty, and freedom of choice. She reminds us not to take it all so seriously. To get off our high horses and just play.

Lauri taught me how to discern, to question, and to go beyond what I thought was possible for myself. Through Lauri, I met a dear friend and fellow cohort in consciousness Megan Bedford. Together the three of us have held each other accountable. To this day we hop on a weekly call to read each other's vibrational fields, call out the stuck points and the misalignments, and help each other come into alignment with the truth of who we are. It's raw, vulnerable, and absolutely glorious. Glorious because of our willingness to see that which prefers not to be seen, slap ourselves in the forehead and go at it again and again until the stuck point resolves and we move beyond it.

Lauri is an *Annie-Get-Your-Gun* personality that holds nothing back. She never hesitates to give me what I call a Universal bitchslap to bring me back into alignment with who and what I am. Most importantly, she is willing to look at her own stuck points and will readily admit to when she is knocking her own head up against the wall. She has taught me that I am not special, just infinite. She has shown me that I am extraordinarily ordinary. Her ability to connect with and bring forth clear and undistorted information from the divine has led the way for me and countless others.

I've captured some of the information she brings forth and

called them Lauri-isms. Any time you see a Lauri-ism, you know the words and wisdom came from her.

HERE'S THE FIRST LAURI-ISM: The world you are in is a wisdom school of misunderstanding to understand. You know you are going into a dream state of experience, a Virtual Reality (VR) room where you sit in a vessel and have an experience. When you create without distortion you know you are in the VR room and you master the vessel. You know you are running the machine with intention and thoughts.

Distorted Creation

Creation goes awry when you forget who you are and create unconsciously. You're powerful and your abilities to create are powerful, but you create with distortion when you don't know who you are or understand that you are the one creating your reality. You create your reality without intention based on negative thoughts and limiting beliefs handed down to you from previous generations or past experiences. You don't consciously discern and choose which thoughts and feelings you would like to experience. You don't create freely from expansion and creativity but in a reactionary and constricted manner with distorted ideas about your worth and value.

You create based on fear, comparison, judgment, guilt, and shame, just to list a few, and you have no idea who you really are. This is called distorted creation. For example, fear is a distorted creation that arises from thoughts and beliefs about past experiences that will most likely never happen again in the future. I'll say that again, fear is based on something that may happen in the future, but rarely does. It's an illusion, a distortion that causes great anxiety. Fear is not real. I mean what is it going to do? Hit you over the head? Fear was created in the VR room. If you knew who you are in truth, you would know that there is nothing to be afraid of.

An unconscious creator forgets who they are and believes themselves to be limited. Most people create unconsciously. They function on autopilot and believe the untrue thoughts, beliefs, and emotions that arise within their field of consciousness, which then in turn creates their reality by default. "I am unworthy" is one of the biggest distortions humanity as a collective has bought into. Guilt and shame are also distortions that arise when we feel we have done something "bad." In fact the whole good/bad, right/wrong paradigm is a complete sham.

Think of the entire universe we live in as one big VR room, often called the Matrix, only it's not like the movie where we try to get out of the Matrix. This matrix we choose to project ourselves into for the experience of it. Most people consider themselves to be Spirit in physical form. From this perspective our Spirit, that exists in non-physical form, agrees to come into the VR room to experience different things for our own growth and evolution and sometimes just for the experience of it. So why wouldn't we want to experience what it's like to play the villain? It truly is a worthy ticket to ride and gives you contrast to get clear on what you like and what you don't like. Every experience is wisdom gained. There is no angry God up in heaven with a white beard judging you for your choices. On the contrary, you are loved unconditionally.

Yes, dear one, you are in a VR room, what I like to call your favorite amusement park. Because there is no judgment you are free to choose any experience you desire. So wherever you have been hard on yourself about your choices, judged what you have done or not done, why not let that go and ask, "What wisdom have I gained? What do I prefer now that I have had all these experiences? And for goodness sake, how can I not take it all so seriously?"

The first and greatest distortion is the illusion that the world you live in is real and the physical body you inhabit is all that you are. You believe yourself to be separate and limited. This gives rise to all other distortions. You fall asleep in the dream. Then what was unlimited freedom, choice, and experience becomes distorted.

Types of Distortions

- **Identity:** In truth you have no identity. Identity only limits that which can never be identified. There is only one consciousness. Individuated, yet one. You could say that there is only one unlimited being exploring the VR room as you and as me. Explore this for yourself; is the conscious awareness that you experience different than the conscious awareness that I experience? Oneness celebrates identity as a beautiful creation knowing in truth we are all part of the One.

- **Death:** When you forget who you are as an unlimited being suddenly there is death. This is not a bad thing. Remember, you came into the VR room to play, to forget and experience death and all the limitations not available to you in the unlimited non-physical, and then to remember who you are. You came to experience the contrast. But when you think death is real and live your life in fear, your view of reality is distorted.

- **Fear:** Fear arose with the belief in death. This came about with the innate need to survive, which was very valid. Today we no longer need to survive the saber tooth tiger, but have kept fear active with the belief that if we take a risk and go outside our comfort zones we might potentially fail, look completely unlovable, or be a bad person. Whew! Talk about distortions! No wonder no one wants to take a risk or make a change! HUGE distortion! You cannot die, you cannot fail, you are more loved than you could ever imagine, and you can never get it wrong!

- **Judgment:** When free will to choose your experience, any experience, was labeled as good and bad it got distorted and judgment arose. Religion and government played roles in creating judgment as a means to control and manipulate. But even in the manipulation there is no good, bad, right, or wrong. Just the experience of it. Even what you might label "bad" serves a purpose. For example, Adolf Hitler played a role for greater clarity. He pushed humanity towards clarity and unity. When people see what they don't want, they are more likely to come together and unite and focus on what they do want. They grow and learn. Humanity has gained much wisdom, much clarity, and experienced a lot of contrast! Just like children grow and learn, so are we as a collective.

- **Guilt and Shame:** These arose along with judgment. If you do what is judged to be wrong or bad, there's a good chance you'll experience guilt. Guilt and shame are not the same. Guilt is I did something bad, and shame is I am bad; both are illusions and distortions created in the VR room by unconscious creators. These typically arise when you've made a choice with which others don't agree. Guilt and shame arise from the good/bad right/wrong paradigm and the birth of should and shouldn'ts.

• **Comparison and Jealousy:** The ideas that you "need to," "have to," or are not enough in any way are also distortions. All creations and expressions are beautiful. Even the shit shows. There is no competition. No one is better than anyone else. There is only choice, preference of experience, and levels of conscious awareness.

The biggest distortion again is the distortion of identity. We think we are the characters we have dropped in to play, not an animating presence articulating it.

Many of us create our realities by default. We don't know we are creators and that we create every moment of every day with our thoughts, choices, and feelings. These things are like beacons to the universe, which replies in kind and sends you more of what you are putting out. You, my dear, are a magnet. Plain and simple. If you are thinking I can't and why try, and you are vibrating in alignment to resignation and apathy, that is what you are magnetizing to you. The universe is a magnet. We know this to be true and science has proven it. We know there are dimensions of unmanifested potential just waiting to respond to your vibration, just like we know atoms and subatomic particles respond to observation and intent.

Let this sink in. I mean really integrate what I am saying here. You are a magnet and you draw things to you via your thoughts and feelings. You are a creation that's been dropped into a VR room and been gifted with the ability to create anything you desire. So this begs the questions, what thoughts are you thinking on a daily basis? Are they positive and uplifting? Joyful and fun? Or are they heavy and serious? Are they unconscious? Or are you fully aware of the thoughts and feelings you are putting out? If you are unconscious, then you are creating by default and have a distorted view of yourself and reality. Your ego or small self is most likely running the show and you may have assumed a victim role, blamed others for your misfortune, and taken on the mantra: "It's not my fault. I can't do anything about it."

If this is the case then your creations are distorted. You look at the world through a lens that is false. And what radiates off you is laced with low energy frequency vibrations, such as fear, guilt, shame, judgment, apathy, resignation, or unworthiness. These are distortions because they are not real. They don't exist. They are thought forms created by man; they are old and outdated. So let's stop it.

Let's break these distortions down even further so you can be super aware of whether they are playing a dominant role in your life. The more aware of them you are, the easier it is to drop them.

Fear: There is no such thing as fear. It's an illusion dreamt up by your thinking mind to keep you safe during the caveman days when we were hunted by predators. But we are no longer hunted today. Today there is nothing to fear but fear itself. Today the mechanism that kept us safe is now a distortion that keeps us from going outside our comfort zones and loving who we are and each other. What do we fear the most? Other distortions such as judgment, unworthiness, rejection, guilt, and shame. We fear what others think. Death is in this list, too. In truth who you are is unlimited, infinite, indestructible, extraordinary, and beyond words. Fear is an illusion.

Judgment: Judgment came about through religions and is used to bring on guilt and shame to keep people in line. I remember sitting in church one day in my youth and hearing that God was a loving God, a forgiving God, and a jealous God. I thought, *What does God have to be jealous of?* It didn't make sense to me then and still doesn't. Who inserted that into the bible was using it to control people from straying to other religions. The idea of "Judgment Day" played its part and weighed heavily on people who thought when they died they would end up at the pearly gates before God and that God would judge them to be worthy and let them in, or unworthy and send them to a fiery everlasting hell. Judgment also came about through the media that promoted that people should look a certain way, have certain things, and if you didn't then you were less than. Judgment and comparison fed into guilt, shame, and the distortion of "I'm not enough." But there is no judgment. Period. God is unconditional love. Love without distortion. Period. Like a mother watching her children hit each other over the head with their toys, God just laughs and shakes his head.

LAURI-ISM: True reality is like God playing with puppets and we are the puppets, but we are given autonomy; we can be whatever we like. God doesn't care what the

puppets do; it just likes to have friends. God compresses its knowing and comes into physical form as you. Then you take a magical mystery trip to find out who you are. Then, when you find out who you are, you get to say what you do.

Your persona is an interface, connected to all that is. When you feel safe to be that which you are, all distortions drop away. So often we compare ourselves to others and find ourselves lacking instead of honoring and accepting our sovereign individual choices. My friend Michelle says that when she meets people, she feels like a puppy dog going up to them with a wagging tail saying, "Hi! What are you experiencing? What have you chosen?" This is acceptance, appreciation, and honoring where each one of us is and what we have chosen in this wild and crazy VR room. When my clients struggle with judgment I have them try on the phrase, "Good on you! I wouldn't choose to have that experience, but good on you!"

Guilt and Shame: Guilt was created when humans set the rules of good and bad, right and wrong, and if you went outside of those parameters, then be damned! But there is no good or bad. There is no right or wrong. We live in a free will universe where we are free to choose any experience we desire and we gain wisdom from it. Imagine yourself for a moment up in heaven and you're with a buddy and your buddy says, "I want to go down and experience what it's like to be a Viking. I want to be big and strong and kill and rape and experience what that's like." And you say, "Okay, I'll go down and I'll be one of those women you rape so I can experience what that's like." It's like cops and robbers. Then when you come sliding back into heaven you have gained wisdom from the experience and you may decide to switch roles. The perpetrator becomes the victim and the victim becomes the perpetrator. No good or bad, right or wrong, just experience for the experience of it and contrast that finetunes what we like and don't like. Guilt and shame are illusions and distortions. Some say it is guilt and shame that keep humans from killing each other until there is no one left. I disagree. I think without guilt and shame what is left is preference and wisdom gained from eons of reincarnating over and over again.

Reality: It's been said that we live in a matrix. That is true. But it is not a matrix we want to escape from. It's a matrix that enables us to experience things from a physical perspective that we couldn't in non-physical. It's an amusement park and you are free to visit the horror house or the merry-go-round or both. You are free to choose your experience without consequence or judgment. Often people have been so driven by guilt and shame of what they should do and shouldn't do that when they finally free themselves, they don't know what to do. I had this experience myself of being so free I had no idea what to choose! This led to a fantastic journey of discovery. You are free to do, be, have, or choose whatever you desire. Sure, there are rules society has created. We live in what is called a collective agreement reality, so there may be consequences to your choice, but you are free. Free to wear what you want, work when you want, eat what you want, and create your reality any way you so choose.

Unworthiness: This distortion also came about through religion and the idea that God is above us, separate from us, not within us. Man had the idea that God is perfect and we are flawed sinners destined to go to hell for doing anything outside of the box of what is considered right or wrong. Unworthiness tells us what we should do or shouldn't do and gives rise to self-doubt. If you do these things then you'll be good enough. If you work hard, be nice, do things for other people, and contribute to society you will go to heaven, and if you don't, you will be judged unworthy and go to hell. Strike the words need to, have to, should, shouldn't, right, wrong, good, and bad from your vocabulary. They are distortions and there are no such things. They are illusions designed to keep you in line and prevent you from discovering the truth of who you are. When I examined the thought, I'm not good enough, I wondered, Who could possibly tell me I was good enough? This made me feel like without this thought of unworthiness I could experience myself as worthy. Then I inquired, am I good enough? Again, I wondered, Who could possibly tell me I was good enough? What this left me with was the feeling that I just am and there is no such thing as worthiness. It's just a bullshit story someone made up that the collective bought into. I am not worthy and I am not lovable are two of the most insidious distortions the collective has bought into.

Apathy and Resignation: These two came about as a result of all the distortions when we were put into the box of what we should do and shouldn't do. Fear, guilt, shame, and judgment came down like a heavy hammer and said, "You are not free!" There was nothing we could do to become good enough, so after working ourselves to the bone trying, much of humanity sank into their couches and gave up. TV, alcohol, food, drugs, and social media became ways to avoid the feelings of "I'll never be good enough, so why try?"

Jealousy and Comparison: These arose when we started seeing what our fellow creators were doing, and instead of getting excited and appreciating what was created or co-creating with them, we had the thought that their creation must be better than ours. Therefore, we must be lacking in some way. Not true! All creation is beautiful in the eyes of the creator.

Separation: The greatest distortion is your inability to perceive yourself as connected to all of existence seen and unseen. There are worlds beyond worlds out there all connected and intertwined in the great tapestry of Oneness. Experience this for yourself. When I say a word, is there any lag between me saying the word and you hearing it? No. It is one field. One consciousness, a consciousness we both share. Can you feel it? When you sit in silence with your beloved can you sense the connection? Something in the space in between? When giving up your belief in separation you lose yourself, only to rediscover yourself.

Unraveling The Distortions

Often distortions take on a life of their own and are embedded deep in our subconscious minds such that we can't seem to dislodge them. We take a crowbar to them and no matter what happens, they don't seem to budge. We think these distortions can't be dismantled. Not true. The crowbar is your awareness. Your willingness to wake up and see the distortions, to shine the light of your awareness onto them is what dissolves them. Your knowing that none of it is real collapses the whole paradigm.

All of these distortions are nothing more than social constructs, dogma, doctrine, a collective agreement of what is so. But it is not so. This is not the truth of the world we live in. Go out in nature and you will see for yourself. There is no judgment when a lion kills a gazelle. There is no guilt or shame as he tears the flesh from its bones. There is no unworthiness found in nature anywhere, and the last thing you would see is two birds sitting on a tree limb comparing worms or lamenting in resignation about how there's just not enough worms today. Nature can teach us many things about the world we live in if only we stop.

STOP.

Look around and wake up. Humanity has been in a collective dream for a long time. The dream of not enough. We've been consuming and consuming, eating more and more, drinking more and more, watching more and more TV, scrolling more and more through social media. More! More! More! All in an effort to get enough or be enough. But enough-ness cannot be found in those things. It can only be found within. It is your birthright just waiting to be discovered.

Today, most of us create our realities unconsciously from the programs embedded into us by our ancestors or the world around us. Our lives are the result of negative thought forms, limiting belief structures, and the untrue story that we are flawed, unworthy humans, not the divine incarnate.

The distortions in our world today were introduced as ideas that when thought over and over became beliefs that became deeply embedded in the personal and collective consciousness. These distortions have limited our abilities to experience the truth of who we are beneath the distortions as extraordinary.

> **REFLECTIVE MOMENT:** Think about this for a moment, who would you be...what would you experience...if fear, guilt, shame, judgment, and feelings of unworthiness were gone?

If you skipped over that reflective moment, stop. Go back. Really ponder it. It's an opportunity to dislodge something from your physical body that no longer serves you. It's also an opportunity to receive an insight or download. All reflective moments in this book are opportunities and I suggest you make the most of them. Play with them, be curious, tap into the young explorer within.

The time to remove these distortions is now. We are no longer children in a sandbox figuring all this out. It is time for a new round of creation, a round of undistorted creation where we are free to go where we want to go, do what we want to do, and express ourselves however we choose. We have gained wisdom from our years of distortions; they have grown old and are no longer needed. It's time to celebrate our individual sovereignty and see what we can create without these distortions. Now that's exciting! It is truly an amazing time to be alive as we herald in this next round of creation and you experience firsthand the extraordinary ordinary you.

This book points to the truth about who you are and what you are beyond distortions. It will show you many ways to remove the distortions and how to create without distortion.

Integration

Today many people are waking up. Some are receiving help through the wisdom of plant medicines; others have been meditating. Both of these communities are undergoing mystical, otherworldly experiences and are coming to know their multidimensional selves. It is more common than ever for someone to experience other dimensions, see the geometric patterns of the VR room, have conversations with deceased loved ones, and experience themselves as subatomic particles, waves, and sound. I have seen people with fibromyalgia, frozen shoulders, low back pain, and neck pain come out of plant medicine experiences completely healed. I have seen men and women who have been sexually abused, physically abused, and emotionally abused see the experience from a new perspective and move on with their life. Many people are connecting with their higher selves and now know themselves as pure unconditional love and Oneness. This is done both with and without plant medicine.

LAURI-ISM: Plant medicine is a natural mechanism to explore the self. It has been culturalized as wrong rather than a natural offering for peace, clarity, and self-discovery.

Plant medicine has been around for centuries. It has been used by indigenous people and shamans worldwide. To utilize plant medicine is a very personal choice. You must turn within and do what feels right for you. I myself have utilized plant medicine as a way to train myself to journey and experience myself without plant medicine, and if that is what you desire you will learn how to do this in the chapters to come. Regardless of the experience, integrating what you experience is very important.

Integration is processing, assimilating, and embodying information that is shown to you. It is putting the information revealed to you on the shelf and pondering it like a Rubik's Cube. It's questioning it, being curious about it, and deciding for yourself what you will keep and what you will discard. Whether in a deep meditation or a plant medicine journey, you can dip into the belly of creation and know experientially that you are not what/who you think you are. Integration is the key. It's one thing to take a dip. It's another thing to hold it here. You can incorporate that information and bring it into your daily life. Integration is the letting go of what you are not and remembering who you are. Integration is a cornerstone throughout this text because it is so very important.

When people integrate their experiences and insights they take the time to let what has been realized settle; they make course corrections in life, let go of what is not serving them and call in more of what does. They increase their conscious awareness, get clarity, and expand their idea of who they are. They take action on the directives or information revealed. Whether that is in the form of releasing a limiting belief, letting go of the story of unworthiness, leaving a relationship that no longer serves them, or healing one that does with honesty and vulnerability. When people integrate, they release low vibrational distortions, such as fear, guilt, and shame, and they magnetize truth, freedom, contentment and love with more ease and clarity. When people integrate they come home to themselves.

It is very common for people to not know what to do with the information gifted to them (whether in meditation or otherwise). People have ineffable experiences and deep knowing of who they are as the divine, yet when no integration is done they come home, go to work, and fall right back into the same habits and patterns. They revert back to their limited humanity. This is what happens when no integration is done.

It is not uncommon for people who have cultivated awareness to have transcendental experiences without plant medicine. The veil between heaven and Earth is thinning and will continue to thin making these experiences available to all. You don't have to do plant medicine to have these types of experiences. But they can help get you started and show the way when they are done with intention and are followed with an integration period to assimilate the information revealed to you.

Integration has a rhythm, a cadence that moves from an experiential insight, knowing, or realization to a period of adjustment where you get used to and embody that new information. You discover a new layer of the self, and take the time to ponder it, be curious about it and get used to it, and integrate it into your daily life. "As above, so below" makes complete sense from an integration perspective.

The Rhythm of Integration

1. Realize a new layer of all of you.
2. You settle and integrate. You get used to it, let your mind accept it, adopt it, embody it.
3. Realize a new layer of all of you.

During the settling period of integration your mind accepts and adapts to the new information and releases the old. This period can feel like a downward slope as everything you thought you knew falls apart so something new can come through. Once adaptation is complete, you are ready for the next experiential knowing or realization. And up that spiral of evolution you go. Taking you ever higher, ever peeling away the layers of what you are not, ever letting go of distortions, taking you ever closer to the essence of that which you are and the things you desire.

Integration is many things. Some people believe integration is taking action afterwards to improve your life. Sometimes this is absolutely the case. But more often than not the directives or revelations suggest just the opposite. Just be. Allow. Surrender. Let go. Receive. Are messages I see in transcripts and journals across the board. Spirit is not usually telling us to leave a relationship or quit our job. Spirit directs us to look inward and face that which needs to be seen and bring forth the love, joy, and fulfillment lying dormant within us.

To me, integration is the tears that fall when you realize a new aspect of yourself. Whether those tears are from the pain and suffering you have caused yourself as you release a distortion, or whether the tears are ones of joy at seeing an aspect of yourself that you hadn't taken into account, or even a glimpse of the true self beyond the stories of who you thought you were. Integration is what happens when an individual is willing to look at themself with openness and curiosity and is courageous enough to face what arises, both the difficult and the unimaginable beauty, and move through it into freedom.

What awaits the individual willing to integrate is freedom. Freedom from the distortions humanity has lived with for eons. Freedom from the lies of not enough-ness, freedom from negative thoughts and limiting beliefs and unruly emotions. With that freedom comes a deep, soft, joyful peace that never leaves. Self doubt is replaced with knowing that who you are can never be measured, can never be explained, can never be limited, and can never be taken away.

The cycle of integration is like riding a roller coaster. At first, moments of insight and awareness come only when the conditions are just right. Maybe you go into the perfect meditation and boom! You find yourself where you never expected to be. Or perhaps some form of plant medicine has given you a glimpse of what lies beyond your ego, and you soar. You see that which is really you and you may leave this realm for a while. This is the up part of the roller coaster that is exciting and open to possibilities. Then, after the meditation is over, or the plant medicine wears off, you come back to this physical world and doubt sets in. Was it real? Did I really have that experience or was it my imagination? Am I really all that, or am I ego? How do I bridge the two so I can navigate this world? Will anyone even believe me that I had this experience? This is the downside of the roller coaster that is filled with fear, self-doubt, confusion, and uncertainty.

Integrating and moving through the downside is a very important part of integration and the point where most people get off the roller coaster, or worse—go for another high without mastering the low. There are gifts in the lows. This is where the distortions are faced, seen for what they are, and released. This is the time when the gunk of the soul is cleansed like Roto Rooter on a gunky pipe, when the ego is lovingly stripped of identity and returned to the faculty it originated as. The downside is when you let the tears fall, when you let the anger rise within you, face it, and feel it move through you and out of you, leaving you strangely at peace.

When you are willing and courageous to be present through the downside, to work out the distortions of what you are not, habits and patterns slowly drop away, old belief systems fade, fear becomes excitement, judgment transforms into acceptance, and guilt and shame become wisdom gained. Wounds heal, the past disappears, and your heart opens. Life becomes easy, joyful, and fulfilling. This is alchemy at its best. This is integration. Integration is also when you allow yourself to experience that which you truly are and let that experience settle within you.

When I work with individuals, I see them move through several phases. At first they must be willing to face that which needs to be seen. The so-called "ugly" parts of themselves they have been avoiding. They face the distortions and begin peeling them away one by one. This is the letting go phase. They face the ego and begin the process of disidentification and true-self discovery. They gain confidence in their ability to handle their emotions; they become the discerner of their thoughts and start mastering the creative process. They then begin to adapt to and integrate the truth of who they are. There are many ups and downs on this road, and for those who are willing to take it, much will be given.

I will be taking you on a very similar journey. This book will help you release that which wants to be released, see that which wants to be seen, and integrate the extraordinary ordinary you. Ordinary because that which lies within you, lies within all.

As you move through this book you will see sections directing you to ponder the information that has been delivered to you. You will then be asked to integrate that information. Do not skip these exercises or pretend that you know them already or blow them off or pay them lip service. That won't get you anywhere. This book is a workbook, designed to be experiential. It contains codes that lie within words designed to trigger a remembering within you. When you feel a truth land within you, sit with it. Be with it, integrate it. If you blow it off or skip over it you may be bypassing an opportunity to come home to yourself.

You will also find that I repeat the same information in different ways throughout this book. This is to help you receive and embody the information presented. When you are reminded of certain concepts at different intervals, in different ways, it makes it easier for the mind to grasp the information and retain it. I recommend you keep a journal to answer the questions throughout this workbook and journal about your realizations to integrate and anchor the information within you.

You will learn how to deal with negative thoughts, limiting beliefs, ego, and emotions, and also how to experience your true self. There are many paths that lead to the discovery of your true self; this is only one. Take what resonates and leave what doesn't. I have found awareness to be the number one and the most effective path. And you don't need plant medicine to cultivate awareness.

You will benefit from integrating your experiences. An experience may come to you as a realization, an experiential knowing, or receiving of information that teaches you something about yourself. It can be astoundingly beautiful and heart wrenchingly painful. Both are equally beneficial to integrate.

I welcome you home to the new world and the new normal as you take your place as a divine being about to shed the layers of what you are not to experience the truth of all that you are.

The Decision to Wake Up

Now before we get started, one thing needs to be very clear. Waking up is a decision. It is a choice. Waking up can be a scary thing because you leave everything that you have known and enter into the unknown, the unfamiliar. This can be shocking. If you never meant to discover yourself as an infinite multidimensional being and suddenly you know that's what you are, it can be quite mind blowing. Many people quickly fall back to sleep so they don't have to confront the enormity of the realization or deal with leaving the familiar behind. So first and foremost understand that while you may want to wake up, your subconscious mind may put up a fight and give you many reasons why waking up may not be such a good idea! It's kind of a big deal.

Let's get really clear about what actually happens when you wake up.

Waking up means you start to realize that who you are is not just the thoughts you ponder about yourself, the beliefs that you hold, and the roles you have played throughout your life. You realize you are not your ego. You may have an identity crisis. If you've asked the question, "Who am I?" and have absolutely no idea...congratulations! You're not going crazy. You're waking up.

Similar to what you do some mornings when you first open your eyes, waking up is not instantaneous. Although that can happen to a very rare few, in general waking up takes the average person many years and many lifetimes to realize they are not the limited personality structure they have identified with, but something different than they've ever imagined themselves to be.

Plant medicine ceremonies, deep contemplative meditation, and cultivating awareness are invaluable at assisting the individual in experiencing themselves outside of all ideas or constructs. They can strip an individual down to nothing, which enables the individual to understand the nature of the void within. When all ideas, identities, or constructs are removed it creates space for true-self discovery.

The good news is you can choose your path to awakening. There are as many paths as there are people. You can wake up gradually simply by cultivating your awareness, you can try a wide variety of plant medicines, you can meditate or do yoga. You can focus on *The Power of Now* like Eckhart Tolle, become a lover of the truth like Byron Katie, or go to an ashram in the East. There is no one way.

I came home by cultivating awareness and that will be emphasized throughout this book. Meditation never seemed to quiet my mind, but I could certainly be aware of my thoughts and surroundings and be curious about them. Cultivating awareness is becoming more and more cognizant of the world around you, the thoughts in your head, the beliefs you hold, and the presence that is you. You become attentive.

What happens when you make the decision to wake up is that any identification with thoughts, beliefs, emotions, or false identities, such as the ego, drop away, and you have an opportunity to experience yourself as you truly are. We can call these moments of self-realization. Then, often as quickly as they come, they recede in the background when your ego or false identity comes back online.

It's crazy to think that you are both a divine particle of God AKA true self, oneness, higher self, divine self, consciousness, or I Am presence (pick what resonates with you most) AND you are an individual AKA the personality self, small self, character self, false self, or ego. How this came to be and how you came to be are mysteries. You, dear one, are the Absolute, the Relative and the Mystery in between, all as One.

Now, the purpose of waking up is not to destroy the ego or personality self. Many people, myself included, have wanted to destroy the ego and go after it with a sledgehammer, which just makes things worse. Trust me, I know. We will talk about the ego in the chapters to come, but for now, know that in the process of waking up your ego returns to the faculty it originated as. It no longer runs the show through chaos, compulsion, knee jerk reactions, or unruly emotions. Instead, it becomes a faithful servant bringing you information. The ego integrates and merges with the divine self. It does not die, but the distortions and identity are removed and it transforms. It's a beautiful melding.

Now, if you have experienced your true self, you know it is indescribable. Words suck. There is just no way anyone could label it. Most of us have a sense that we are more than just our physical bodies. Many of us have moments of clarity when the rest of the world falls away and we experience deep peace and a sense of our inner being.

> **REFLECTIVE MOMENT:** Imagine for a moment that you are not your body or the label of husband or wife or artist or entrepreneur. That all the labels and identities you have worn throughout your life fall away. Let all negative thoughts or beliefs about yourself go too. What's left? Be curious. Does it feel limited in any way? Does it feel in need of anything? Are you really separate?

Please understand that you are an unlimited and infinite being who has decided to forget who you are in order to experience what it would be like to be limited, and to wake up and experience yourself anew. How cool is this?

This brings us to some options. If you decide to wake up, you have two choices:

- You can ascend and do an "Oh my God! I know who I am!" and peace out and leave your physical body behind, because it really is that amazing.

OR

- You can be on the cutting edge and decide that you want to wake up AND stay in physical form. This is called embodied ascension and is now a possibility for all humanity.

To embody your divinity means that the physical body increases in vibrational frequency from that of density and distortion to one that is less dense and divine. This doesn't mean that you float away, it means that every cell in your body knows who you are and what you are and you have a new vehicle to play with. Someone once told me that Jesus transformed his physical form into light in front of his disciples. And he said in John 14:12, and I paraphrase, "All that I can do, you can do and more."

Think about this for a moment. Never before have we as a species had so much support, so much guidance, or such a big increase in our vibrational fields. Change is happening on the planet faster than ever before. The more people wake up, the more they break ground for those who follow. What you do on behalf of yourself during the awakening process you do for all mankind. This is like the four-minute-mile that no one thought could be broken. Then when Roger Bannister broke the record, others believed they could too, and it became the new normal. Embodied divinity may soon be the new normal.

How exciting is this!

We can explain waking up in many different ways:

- From the vibrational perspective we could describe it as increasing our frequency from low to high. Vibrations refer to the oscillating and shaking movement of atoms and particles caused by energy within you. Frequency, which is measured in hertz (Hz) units, is the rate at which those vibrations and oscillations occur. Frequencies are used to determine and differentiate vibrational patterns. The planet and each human has his or her own unique vibrational pattern and frequency that we use to create and attract what we desire. As you come into alignment with, and claim yourself as divine source, you transition from the lower frequencies to the higher frequencies.

• We can also explain waking up from an emotional perspective. There are low vibrational frequency emotions that give you a certain experience, such as anger, fear, anxiety, depression, self doubt, and frustration, and you have high vibrational frequency emotions that give you experiences of contentment, knowing, gratitude, joy, and love. And a wide variety of vibrational experiences in between. These have been measured by science. We can increase our frequency or decrease our frequency by choosing thoughts and setting intentions that bring about certain emotions. When you wake up, you leave the distortions behind and align with the frequencies of unconditional love, joy, peace, and wonder. Emotions can be excellent guides that let you know where you are in the awakening process.

• We could describe waking up as a transition of beliefs. You trade in beliefs of yourself as a separate limited being for your true identity as an unlimited, infinite being connected to all things. Oneness. Union. You see yourself as a strand in the tapestry of life and how one strand affects all other strands and adds to its depth, richness, and glory.

• We could also describe waking up as a process where you cultivate awareness. As you cultivate awareness you let go of what you are not, and acclimate and explore with curiosity consciousness itself.

- Waking up could be the process of removing distortions gradually to peel away the layers of what you are not, eventually revealing what you are.

- Waking up can consist of many moments of realization. Realization comes to individuals who are open to alternative possibilities, perceptions, downloads, or insights and knowings that come in a variety of ways. Moment by moment and realization by realization they gradually trust in the unknown and the unfolding until they are in their knowing of who and what they are in truth.

Again, there are many ways to wake up. Trauma, for example, can cause people to wake up instantly, but more often waking up rarely happens all at once. It can be a slow process.

What Awakening May Look Like

- As you relinquish the false self and acclimate to the higher frequencies and know yourself as infinite and connected, you will be required to make choices to bring your environment into alignment with the divine self or to stay in the lower frequencies of fear, lack, and limitation.

- It may come as an experiential knowing that you are not who you thought you were. Then as you become more aware of your thoughts and beliefs, and how they limit you, you become more willing to explore what exists beyond them. At first, you may catch a negative thought after the fact. Then as you continue to cultivate awareness, you may catch yourself in the middle of the thought. Then, you may catch yourself just before the thought arises in your awareness. This is another way you can measure your progress.

• Patterns that used to manifest as emotional triggers will get less intense and less frequent, fading into the background and becoming more and more subtle, requiring more and more awareness to dissolve them.

• The degree to which you assume your true identity may fluctuate because you don't maintain consciousness. You may be conditioned to respond to certain things in certain ways based on old patterns, paradigms, social constructs, and old belief systems. It may take time to unknow these things.

• The ego will usually come out kicking and screaming once you decide to wake up because it thinks it will be the death of it. Again, the ego does not die; it transforms back to the faculty it originated as and works with you in partnership. The more you work with the ego by thanking it, loving it, and gently removing identity from it, the less active it becomes.

• You gradually trade control for trust. Instead of micromanaging everything you let go and trust that source has you. You still take action, but the action you take is inspired action—which is taking action that feels like it's compelled by your soul—and the results of your action produce higher quality results. You trade fear for faith and low quality action for high quality action that arises from your being.

• You experience more and more moments of true self. You begin to align to the source of all things. You may call the source God, Mohammed, Love, Divine, Infinite, Oneness,

Universe, Knowing, Awareness, Consciousness, All That Is; there are many names. For the sake of this book we will use many of these knowing they point to the same thing.

• When the false self decides something, it is based on the limitations of the past and the only thing it can conjecture are things that it already knows, which is very limiting. As you awaken, you let your past drop away and spend more moments in the now— exploring, playing, and just being. You take inspired action that lights you up.

• Integration is when you have aligned with divinity as true self and know your physical self to be a coherent articulation of the divine in expression without distortion. It is a union. You navigate life as an integrated whole and are being directed by your higher knowing. It's like you as consciousness get to ride this really cool physical vehicle that enables you to talk, taste, touch, feel, and experience the world around you. That, dear one, is magical, wondrous, and extremely joyful!

Aligning with your inherent divinity requires courage and a leap of faith. The certainty of the known is left behind to realize that which is beyond the known. This means leaving the comfortable self you have created behind—the one who likes this, disagrees with those people, judges this, is ashamed of those things. Self-realization comes to those who are willing to release expectations of what should be for what is.

It may be helpful in your decision-making process to note that many people associate being holier than thou, strict, or pious with awakening or enlightenment. Not so. Others think life will be boring, bereft of any fun, emotions, or other traits. I certainly did. Rest assured, the divine does have a sense of humor and life as an awakened being is never dull.

Know that if you are a writer, you will continue to create. If you are a business owner, you will continue on. But you will do these activities from a higher level of consciousness that brings more quality and joy to the experience or creation. You don't have to change your career or your life's work unless you are called to do so. Whatever you choose to do for a living will give you a sense of truth that your work is right for you and who you are and your gifts.

Some of you may decide that this is the life where you remember who you truly are, and go forth on a fantastic journey toward union. Others may say, "I understand the idea, but no thank you. Maybe in my next life I will trust enough to take the journey." No one way is right or wrong, better or worse. We all take the journey at some point.

So what do you say? Do you choose to participate in the great unknowing? Are you ready to take the journey?

If you are ready to move forward, turn the page.

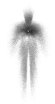

CHAPTER 1

THOUGHTS, PART ONE

You're still here.

Congratulations on your decision to wake up! You have magnetized this book into your hands and that is an indicator that you are indeed in the process of waking up. Take a moment to honor yourself and your decision.

Good.

Now, let's start this journey by tackling the first challenge to waking up. Let's start with your thoughts. Like any hero's journey of self-realization you will encounter hurdles, and your thoughts are one of them. As Robin Sharma says, "The mind is a wonderful servant, but a terrible master."

Thoughts play a critical role in determining whether you expand and evolve beyond your perceived limitations or fall back into your old habits, negative mental patterns, and false identities. The thoughts you choose are how you create your reality, so knowing how to navigate and master your thinking mind is essential.

As you become more and more aware of thoughts and the role they play in creating your life and reality, the more you realize how many thoughts have slipped by you without even questioning them. In the beginning you may feel like thoughts are uncontrollable and are constantly beating you up. Thoughts, when you first become aware of them, can be overwhelming, judgmental, aggressive, and downright mean. Thoughts can be a real bitch.

When I work with individuals I see them move through several phases: At first they must be willing to face what needs to be seen and deal with it. The so-called "ugly" parts of themselves they have been avoiding: the negative self-talk, self-hatred, the pain, sadness, anger, and sorrow they have been avoiding. Once they realize facing these things will not kill them, they begin to unwind the negative thought patterns and release stored emotions one by one. They face the ego and begin the process of disidentification and true-self discovery. Then they gain confidence in their abilities to handle their emotions; they become the discerners of their thoughts, the chooser of thoughts, and start mastering the creative process.

To become the conscious creator of your life you MUST become the chooser of your thoughts. To become the chooser of thoughts, you MUST cultivate awareness. It is awareness that dissolves the thoughts you don't want and enables you to choose the ones you do want. When you cultivate awareness you literally watch a thought come and go without getting hooked by it or feeling any attachment to it. You watch it dissolve right before your eyes. No thought can withstand the power of your pure awareness. Not one.

The following chapters will walk you through exactly how to master your mind and choose the thoughts that arise within your field of consciousness. Eventually difficulty will give way to ease, the highs and lows of the emotional roller coaster will even out, drama will be eliminated from your life, and you will reside more and more in a place of no thought.

Let's tap into some tools that may be beneficial in helping you identify and release thought patterns that no longer serve you. Simple, practical, and scientific ways of dealing with thoughts will be presented so that you may better understand them. But first let's learn more about this faculty called the mind and the thoughts it brings forth.

Thoughts Create Reality

Thoughts are what create your reality. Period. You may have heard this over and over and probably thought, yeah right. But it is true. Science has shown us that what we think about really becomes what we bring about. Olympic and world-class athletes know very well when they use their imagination and direct their thoughts and visualize themselves performing an event and winning, it increases the potential of them actually achieving first place. Numerous studies prove those who direct and choose their thoughts and visualize the end result are most likely to achieve it. Olympic medalist Michael Phelps talks frequently about how he used visualization in order to achieve the goal of becoming one of the world's best swimmers. (You can watch the visualization techniques Phelps used on YouTube.)

Let's look at what goes on in your head on a regular basis. Are the thoughts that come to you every day generally positive and uplifting? Or negative and outside of your control? Write the thoughts that come to you daily down.

Now look at your life and compare it to these thoughts. Is your life generally positive and uplifting? Or negative and outside of your control? They match, don't they?

Let's go a bit deeper and explore some examples of how thoughts create reality. For example, if you think money is bad, you probably don't have much of it. If you think you can't do anything more than work a low paying job, that's probably your reality. If you think you don't have time for spiritual work, then I don't have time is most likely your reality.

Have you said (or thought), "I just can't do it, or I'm not good enough?" This type of thinking keeps people separate from who they really are and what they can do. These are just thoughts that have arisen, not who you are. When you buy into these thoughts and believe them to be true it creates a false reality regarding who you are.

Yup. You are the creator of your life, and you do so with your thoughts. Let me say that again because it is the foundation of everything we are discussing here: You are a powerful creator and you create with your thoughts. So this begs the questions: What are you creating? And is it to your liking?

Regardless of whether you are creating consciously or unconsciously, or how uncomfortable it might be to take responsibility for your creations, now is the time to accept your power and clean up any messes that were made while you were asleep.

When you see that you are not the thoughts with which your mind thrashes you, but the observer of those thoughts, you begin to untangle from them. So from now on, assume the role of the conscious observer—not the unconscious reactor—and start actively observing and releasing thoughts that no longer serve you. This can be done as easily as flicking something from your shoulder or as difficult as pushing a two-ton truck uphill. The choice is yours. I recommend taking the easy path. What is the easy path? Cultivating awareness. It will raise you above thought. I'll show you how in just a bit.

But first, let's take a deeper look into your mind and learn how thoughts work.

According to Dr. Joe Dispenza, thoughts are what create our moods, our temperaments, and even our personalities. Dr. Dispenza's research has shown how thoughts create your personality, or who you think you are. He explains:

1. First your mind creates a thought. When you have that thought over and over and buy into it, it becomes a belief. Those thoughts and beliefs create a MOOD.

2. When you experience this mood over and over and over, the mind can't tell the difference between what is imagined and what is real, so it becomes a TEMPERAMENT.

3. The more you experience this new temperament, it becomes ingrained into your mind until your brain associates it with the pattern of you. It becomes your PERSONALITY!

REFLECTIVE MOMENT: This begs the Question: How have your thoughts contributed to your moods, temperament, and personality?

Look at your daily repetitive thoughts and your personality. Do you see a correlation?

How have your daily thoughts contributed to the quality of your life?

What thoughts would you like to let go of?

What thoughts would you like to bring into your daily life to create a different reality?

Turn those new thoughts into a brief mantra. For instance, when I was struggling with thoughts of unworthiness I wanted more peace so I used the mantra: Peace. Trust. Truth. Knowing. Let go. And Love. I repeated these words several times a day, especially when the thought pattern I can't or Who am I to do that? arose. Some days I really needed trust and other days peace really helped me quiet my mind. Just by saying the word "Peace" my body responded. Just by saying the words "Let go" my mind relaxed. This helped me deactivate the old pattern and create a new one. Words are like codes that can trigger a relaxation effect on the body, which helps us release and let go.

What mantra will you create that will help unwind your old pattern? Keep it brief and easy to remember. Choose words that feel good.

Use this mantra daily whenever you feel a negative thought pattern arise. Use the code to interrupt current patterned ways of thinking and to create new ones. Think of it as de-programming and reprogramming your system.

Thoughts Create Your Personality

The role thoughts have in creating the personality you call "You" is immense, which is a very good reason to be sure you are choosing the right ones.

To be clear, your personality is made up of your thoughts, beliefs, perceptions, and interpretations. This is what determines how you respond to the world around you. For instance,

- If you fall off the swing and cry as a child and interpret swings to be bad or dangerous, fear of swings may become a part of your personality.

- If you fall off a swing and laugh, get back on, and try to swing higher, love of swings may become a part of your personality.

Both scenarios are the same event: falling off the swing. How you perceive and interpret that fall determines what type of personality you create. One event. Two possible personalities. Cool, huh?

Now it's important to point out that you are not your personality. Your personality is the culmination of how you were raised, how your parents or guardians influenced you, and how your mind perceived and interpreted certain events and the world around you. These things are what created the personality you call you. But that's not you. That is just the personality structure you think is you. It's the character on the stage of life that the divine within you articulates, and you can change the character whenever you choose.

This may seem like I'm hitting you with a lot right out of the gate, but it really is time for the illusion to end and for humanity to wake up, so I won't be mincing too many words. However, you can implement my suggestions at your own pace. So feel your way through this text and stop if you feel overwhelmed and need a break to integrate the information.

Okay, back to the point I was making: you are an articulation of the divine. To understand who and what you really are, let's start peeling away the layers of what you are *not*. This will take you to the heart of what/who you really are. Let's continue our tour of thoughts and learn more about what we should have been taught in fifth grade.

Your Brain is an Organ

Your brain is an organ just like your heart and your lungs.

- Your heart is an organ that beats. From the time you are born until the day you die your heart will beat. That is what it does. You have no control over it.

- Your lungs are organs that breathe. That's what they do. From the time you take your first breath until the day you exhale your final, your lungs inhale and exhale.

- Your brain is just like your heart and lungs, only instead of beating or breathing, it houses the mind which thinks. And like the heart and lungs, you have no control over it. It runs your other organs and brings you information all day. You can't control it, but you can choose what information you accept and what information you reject, and it will adapt. The mind is trainable.

The Birth of the Ego

The mind is actually a faculty designed to bring you information. Like your eyes, ears, nose, and mouth bring you information, the mind brings you information in the form of thoughts, which become beliefs and trigger emotions. Your job is to be the discerner of the information that comes to you and consciously choose what feels true and right to you.

This faculty of the mind, when left to its own devices, creates a false identity called the ego. Instead of you as the observer discerning which thoughts you accept into your reality and which ones you reject, you decide to take a little nap and let the ego choose. The ego doesn't have much common sense. It just wants to keep you safe. So it accepts all information that comes in as true. The next thing you know you are a bundle of negative thoughts and limiting beliefs like I'm not good enough that you never discerned or actively chose.

You may identify with thoughts like I'm not lovable, I can't, or I don't know enough, which then become beliefs, which then become a part of a personality structure that you think is you.

But those things are not you, not by a long shot. They just slipped past your discernment.

Just like you would not identify with your breath or your heartbeat, it doesn't make sense to identify with or even believe the thoughts that arise within your mind. Just like you use your mouth as a faculty to discern what you will and will not put into it, you must now use your awareness to discern what thoughts you will and will not put into your reality.

This is why it is so important to cultivate awareness.

When you are aware of the thoughts the mind brings you, it gives you the opportunity to redirect the mind and have it retrieve something better. You can do this by saying, "Nope. That is not helpful. Get me something better."

LAURI-ISM: Quandary is the mind finding its place. When the mind isn't directed, it will bring you all kinds of random information based on the past or collective dogma or doctrine. Telling it to find new information helps it dial into new information from the universe. Literally tell it to stop with the shit and bring you something better. The mind is the bringer, you're the receiver. It's up to you to direct it. It's a Google system that brings information to you. It is the natural order of receiving information so be sure to thank it for bringing

expedient answers into form.

MEDITATION: To cultivate awareness, sit quietly and be very still in the room you are in. Imagine you just heard a sound outside and it startled you so your senses are on high alert. Listen for sounds, the creaking of a wall, the ticking of a clock, the hum of a fan. Bring your awareness to your body and where it is located in the room. Feel your chest rise on the inhale and fall on the exhale. Can you feel your heart beat in your chest? Do not close your eyes and go inward or disappear. Stay relaxed and alert. Wait for a thought to arise in your field of awareness. When a thought arises, watch it come and watch it go. Don't judge what arises. Get used to being in the role of the aware discerner. Choose a negative thought and feel how your body responds. Then direct your mind to choose a positive thought and feel that. Then, simply watch your thoughts come and go without attachment so you can get a feel for yourself as the aware presence. Do you see how you as the aware presence is the chooser? The creator of your reality? Wouldn't it be wise to choose thoughts that bring forth feelings that are enjoyable?

INTEGRATE: Stop here. Do not continue on until you have answered the questions and done the exercises and meditations. Take notes about any insights you've had or revelations to fully integrate what has been revealed to you. I find writing in a journal to be very helpful. I will write down information that I really want to embody. It enables me to engage with the information differently and helps to integrate the material at a deeper level. Then when I want to review what I want most to remember I can thumb through my journal.

CHAPTER 2

THOUGHTS, PART TWO

Quick Recap: So far you have learned that thoughts create reality and the personality you call you so it's important to choose them consciously. You discovered that the brain is an organ that houses the mind which thinks and you can train it to bring you new information instead of repeating the same old information. When you identify with thoughts the ego/ false identities are born. You have done a meditation designed to cultivate awareness of yourself as an aware presence and choose thoughts according to how they make you feel. Hopefully you experienced yourself as the aware discerner and chooser.

Let's continue our exploration of thoughts.

Don't Resist Your Thoughts

Because you have no control of the thoughts that arise in your awareness, it is important not to push them away or pretend they don't exist. The more you resist your thoughts, the more you will struggle. Trust me on this. In the beginning I resisted my thoughts and tried to push them away and it just made things worse. Resisting your thoughts is like resisting the beating of your heart. Resistance is futile.

When you step back into your role as the discerner, false identities or ego structures come to the surface to fight. This can be marked by ups and downs, depression, self-doubts, and many overwhelming emotions. It may seem like you are completely out of control of your thoughts and they can really beat you up. You may feel unable to focus on any thought for even a short period of time or to direct your thoughts. This is very normal. You are in the uncomfortable beginning phases of retraining your mind. The good news is it gets easier as you move along and you retrain it by always asking for something better.

Many people have blazed the road ahead of you and have cultivated awareness, stepped back into their roles as discerners, the choosers and creators of their realities and have awakened to who they are beyond their thoughts. As they dissolve thought patterns and bust beliefs both individually and collectively, it becomes easier for you. What they do on behalf of themselves contributes to the collective field and becomes available to you. We are one, remember? So take heart. We are all on the same team. It is now easier than ever to cultivate awareness and assume your place as a free and conscious chooser of your thoughts and therefore your reality.

Some Thoughts Are Not Yours

Some thoughts that arise in your field of awareness may not even be yours. We have what is called a collective mind or a collective consciousness. A collective consciousness is the set of shared beliefs, ideas, and moral attitudes which operate as a unifying force within society. It is a shared understanding of social norms, an agreed reality.

Storytime: Once upon a time humanity decided to work together collectively to create some rules and structure so people would stop hitting each other over the head with rocks and killing each other. They sat around a campfire and made up some rules that everyone agreed to follow. They created a container for these shared thoughts and beliefs and called them the collective consciousness. Now these beings weren't that advanced so they created rules like "light is good" and "dark is bad" because if you went against the rules and went out at night or went outside of the safety zones you might die. "The world is not safe" was one of the first beliefs added to the collective.

As the society matured and became teenagers, other rules like, "you have to work hard to get ahead," "money is bad," "it's important to look good and not look bad," and "in order to belong you must conform" were added to the first beliefs. Then "I'm not good enough" and "I'm not loveable"—two of the most insidious collective beliefs—were added to the pot. Emotions were labeled bad; you definitely don't want to feel those because they are not pleasant. Alcohol, food, TV, and social media were great and very acceptable ways to avoid emotions. Anything that felt good was good, and anything that felt bad was bad. Fear was a motivating factor in creating the collective consciousness and everything was founded on fear, judgment, guilt, and shame. The collective consciousness was designed to remind humans about the rules and beliefs they had all agreed upon. So every once in a while a thought or belief may pop into your conscious mind to remind you of this collective agreement.

Today, the collective consciousness is very outdated and in serious need of an upgrade because the community has matured into adulthood. We now face the task of cleaning it up. So some humans have come together and decided to step back into the seat as the observer of the thoughts that arise within their individual field of consciousness and decide if a thought or belief serves the community or individual or not. If it serves the higher good, it is kept. If it does not, it is released. Individuals today are getting really good at discerning which thoughts are theirs and which thoughts are from the collective and the collective consciousness is changing.

Family lineage and ancestral patterns handed down through generations are dismantled this way. Love is replacing fear, acceptance is replacing judgment, and appreciation for the unique and diverse differences among us is replacing comparison. "The world is not safe" is becoming "The world is safe." "In order to belong you must conform" is becoming "You are free to express and be." "I'm not good enough" and "I'm not loveable" are becoming ridiculous, and emotions are now valuable indicators that tell us where we are with ourselves.

LAURI-ISMS: "You have to work hard" is becoming "Work is doing what you love and receiving in kind for it." "Money is bad" is becoming "Money is the degree which you allow yourself to be loved by the universe."

As society masters transmuting the old into new, it is now fun to alchemize and change the collective agreements. More joy, more love, and more acceptance are entering the world. Experiences of the past as perpetrator and victim are losing their meaning and are now being realized as wisdom gained from experience. The community is now coming into balance and harmony. Yes, old systems are falling down so that the new can come through. While this looks like destruction, and it is, it is simply creating space for free expression and undistorted creation.

> **REFLECTION MOMENT:** The old paradigm is clearly crumbling and those who hold onto it will have a more difficult time than those who are willing to adapt and change. Which one are you? Are you willing to let go of the old paradigm of fear, judgment, guilt, and shame? Are you willing to see these distortions and let them go? Who would you be and what would you experience without these distortions in your life?

You Are Not Your Thoughts

Just because your mind formulates a thought, that is not who you are. You are not your thoughts. For example, many people have been exposed to the thought or belief that they are not good enough and believe it to be who they are: individuals who are not good enough. But this isn't true. It's just a thought or belief that they bought into and identified with.

When you identify with "I am not good enough" (and believe it) a false mind-made self filled with suffering and pain is created. In other words, when you buy into the story that you are not good enough, a false aspect of your personality has been born.

When you dis-identify or disassociate from "I am not good enough" and don't believe it, a space is created for you to discover what/who you are. Disassociating from thoughts creates space for awareness of the true self to arise. You become the observer of your thoughts, not the thoughts themselves.

Again, just because your mind thinks something doesn't mean it's true. Always ask for something better.

Your Thoughts Want to Protect You

While the thoughts coming from the mind may try to sabotage you and may sound very mean, they are not unfriendly aspects of your personality. They just want to keep you safe from failure, judgment, or discomfort. When you buy into a thought, it will often try to keep you safe by persuading you not to take action. For instance, "Don't speak up and share your perspective. People might not agree and you could be rejected." Or "don't change your lifestyle and exercise. Life won't be any fun."

In other words, stay stagnant; it's safe here. You remain safe, protected, comforted, and in the same old unfulfilling routine and belief system. Your need for certainty and security is met. But in staying safe, you miss out on your dreams and may never see what's waiting for you beyond the perceived safety. While your thoughts want to keep you safe and are very well intentioned, in reality they create way more suffering than they prevent.

Most Thoughts Are Not True

In 2005, the National Science Foundation published an article regarding research about human thoughts. The average person has between 12,000 to 60,000 thoughts each day. Of those, 80 percent are negative and untrue, and 95 percent are exactly the same repetitive thoughts as the day before. Let's say that again. Up to 80 percent of the thoughts that spontaneously arise in our awareness every day are mostly negative and untrue. In addition, 95 percent of them are repetitive.

Wow! This accounts for the fact that so many of us do the same things day after day after day and get caught up in patterns of repetition. Is it any wonder breaking free from old habits and patterns and identity structures is difficult. We've been on autopilot and the navigation system is severely outdated.

Thoughts Are Not Real

Thoughts aren't tangible. Can you hold a thought in your hand? Can you prove it exists? For example, when a thought appears, if you pay no attention to it, if you don't buy into it, it simply disappears without a trace. It arises in awareness and disappears in awareness.

The only way a thought becomes your reality is when you choose to embrace it, when you believe it.

MEDITATION: Every morning before you jump out of bed, become aware of your thoughts and mood upon awakening. If they are negative and outside of your control, spend 10 minutes doing a gratitude rant about some of the things in your life that you are grateful for. Then do a love rant about the things you love and enjoy in life so that you are consciously choosing to start your day feeling positive. I mean, if you're going to create a story, why not create a good one that makes you feel happy?

Your Thoughts Create Your Life

Even though thoughts aren't tangible, your thoughts still create your life.

• For instance if you have the thought, I can't choose my thoughts, and you believe it or buy into it, that concept becomes a part of your personality. You've mistaken the thought for who you are and identify as someone who can't choose their thoughts and this becomes your reality.

• However, if you have the thought, I can choose my thoughts, and you believe or embrace that, it becomes a part of your personality and you identify as someone who can choose your thoughts and this becomes your reality.

Which reality is real? The story of I can? Or the story of I can't? *(The answer is whichever you choose to believe.)*

We create our own reality by choosing the thoughts we identify with. In fact, "I am not good enough," "I am not lovable," and "I can't" or "I don't have time" are the biggest lies society has collectively bought into. These thoughts have created very painful realities for many people.

Whether or not we believe a thought depends on whether or not it becomes true or real for us. Every human has their own personal reality based on their perceptions and interpretations of the world around them. No two humans have ever had the exact same experience.

In order for us to find our own truths and choose our own realities consciously, we need to be able to discern whether a thought is true or not for us. Not our parents, not our partner, not the collective, but for us as sovereign individuals.

Imagine what would happen if every one of us decided right now not to let a thought go by without discerning whether it was true and choosing what feels good? Pretty powerful stuff, huh?

So let's make this dream of being conscious creators a reality. Let's do The Work.

The Work

In her book, *Loving What Is*, Byron Katie has developed a

phenomenal way to discern a thought's truth. She calls it "The Work," which consists of four questions and a turnaround. The four questions are:

1. Is it true?
2. Can you absolutely know that it's true?
3. How do you react, what happens, when you believe that thought?
4. And who would you be without the thought?

The turnaround is a way of experiencing the opposite of the thought that one is believing. For example, the thought "My husband should listen to me," can be turned around to "I should listen to my husband," "I should listen to myself," and "My husband shouldn't listen to me."

Using this methodology you can ponder how each turnaround might be "just as true" as the original thought.

The only way to know The Work is just to do it.

Write down the top negative, self-defeating thoughts, or limiting beliefs your mind likes to thrash you with. Feel free to get petty and just dump it all out.

Now, hold those thoughts up to some scrutiny. Look at the first thought and explore with curiosity these questions:

1. Is what you have written down true? Try not to get too analytical about this question. This is an experiential exercise of finding the truth, not a mental exercise, so *feel* your way through it.

2. Because the mind can be devious, we need to ask this a second time: "Can you ABSOLUTELY know that it's true?" Don't get caught up in the truth-ness of it. If you wrote down, "I am fat," ask, "What does being fat mean to me?" and you will get at the heart of your self-defeating thought or limiting belief.

   Once you discern if the thought is true or not, keep going. Don't skip over these last two questions. They are the best part!

3. How do you feel when you believe or think that thought?

REFLECTIVE MOMENT: Really take your time here. Who would you be without all those thoughts you wrote down? True or not true, who would you be? What would you experience?

Go through this process slowly and deliberately with each of your negative thoughts or limiting beliefs and watch them fade away.

There's one more element to The Work, it's called the turnaround. This involves projection, judgment, and opposition. While we like to think we don't judge, we all do it and often. What we judge in others is usually a reflection of what we judge in ourselves. It can also be an indicator that tells us when we are being judgmental. Sometimes it is hard to see those things about ourselves that don't want to be seen, but in order to move beyond them it is necessary.

Example of a Turnaround: He is a jerk becomes I am a jerk, or he is not a jerk. I am not good enough becomes I am good enough. I can't do this becomes I can do this.

Be gentle with yourself and what you discover. Have compassion. After all, you've been unconscious. What can you expect?

What turnaround is available to you? Think in oppositions or redirect the thought back at yourself in a different way. Ask your mind to bring you something more, something in alignment with truth.

INTEGRATE: Do not move on until you have fully integrated the information in this chapter.

Sit with it for a moment and ponder what you have learned. Be curious about it, journal about it, and get used to it. Put sticky notes on your fridge to remind you of the truth you discovered. Return to the information in this book several times as you go about your day, your week, and your month to incorporate this new information into your life.

The more you do The Work and pay attention to your thoughts, noting whether they are true or not, the more you'll experience brief moments of *no thought*, where you can sense your inner being beyond thought. The more you do this, the more you dis-identify with thoughts, the more you sense your true nature, your true being, who you are beneath the chaos and compulsion of your thinking mind, you find you.

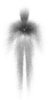

CHAPTER 3:

THOUGHTS, PART THREE

Quick Recap: In the last chapter you learned it is important not to resist thoughts. Resistance is futile. But you can redirect them and ask for something better. You discovered that some thoughts may sneak into your awareness that arise from the collective, things we have all agreed upon that are very outdated, like the whole idea that we are unworthy or unlovable beings. We covered that you are not your thoughts and identifying with them creates false identities. While thoughts want to protect you and most are not true, they do create your life so it is wise to choose them consciously. You learned how to do The Work to determine a thought's truth and you learned a gratitude meditation.

Let us continue our journey through the world of thoughts, and learn more about how to direct and utilize this thing called the mind.

Choosing Your Thoughts

As you unwind and let certain thoughts go, practice redirecting the mind to where you would like it to go. Choose thoughts based on how they make you feel. For example, let's say you wake up and the first thing that comes to you is, Oh no, this is going to be a shitty day. Powerful creator that you are, this is probably not the best way to start your day.

So simply choose the thoughts you would like to experience upon waking. Simple. Yes. Easy? Sometimes and sometimes not so much.

Some mornings you may wake up and it is very easy to direct your thoughts and think about what you are grateful for and how you would like the day to unfold. My favorite morning mantra is, "Thank you! Thank you! Thank you for this human body that lets me taste, touch, see, hear, and speak! Whoa! God in physical waking up! Thank you for this comfortable bed, the roof over my head, the food in my belly, and my ability to choose my reality. Today I choose joy. Today I choose to meet what arises with an open heart and an open mind. Today I choose to not take life seriously and trust I am where I am meant to be."

Somedays directing my thoughts is anything but easy. I used to wake up and my ego wouldn't have anything to do with anything positive. "What! Feel good for no good reason? Hell no." Pissy Patty is what I called my ego and some days she was a force to be reckoned with. "I don't want to," "Screw this," "It's too hard," "Maybe tomorrow," and "I don't have time" were her favorite phrases. And redirecting my thoughts and asking for something better felt like moving mountains.

Be very compassionate with yourself as you go through the letting go process. Be compassionate with your ego and remember that its intentions really are to keep you safe. It just doesn't know any better. When the ego acts up and starts thrashing you, put your hand on your heart and thank it for its positive intentions and continue to let go of the information it brings you and ask for something better. Eventually you will love this faculty and how it has helped create the unique personality structure called you. Love it, don't fight it, be gentle and compassionate as you work with the ego.

I remember one day I had succeeded in redirecting my thoughts and pushed through Pissy Patty's objections, I felt like I had won a huge battle! In my mind I stood triumphantly over her and cheered myself on...until she slapped me back down again. This went back and forth for some time until I stopped fighting her and got better and better at thanking her and moving on with my day. The less attention I gave her, the more she receded in the background. Now, I know she is just a remnant of an old pattern unwinding.

Choosing your thoughts is an act of self-governance. It's an act of creation. When you say, "I suck," you indeed suck. When you say, "I choose to be happy," you are happy. Thoughts become words that inform and encode belief structures that become your world and who you are. It is a beautiful thing. I have heard it said before that we are so free that we can imprison ourselves with the negative thoughts and limiting beliefs we buy into. I certainly found this to be true.

LAURI-ISM: Thoughts are consciousness where you can choose from the menu presented to you like library shelves filled with thoughts. When you choose the top shelf but are vibrating at the lower, you have to rise in vibration to meet your choice.

You can't just say I choose love and be vibrating in doubt. If you choose love, you must bring yourself into vibrational alignment by *feeling* love. Ask the mind to bring you information regarding love and actually feel it. Be curious about it. Explore it. Different feelings have different frequencies so when you choose a thought consciously feel the result of your choice.

For the longest time I chose thoughts of joy, love, and fulfillment, but those things weren't manifesting in my life. It wasn't until Lauri told me I wasn't aligning to the feelings, that I was just talking and getting nowhere. That's when it hit me like a ton of bricks. Doh! Yes, if I choose love, I have to feel love to be in alignment with that choice. Got it!

Here's a simple and quick primer on how you create via thoughts:

- Choice

- Self-awareness

- Vibrational alignment

You choose the thought, become aware of where you are vibrating within, and bring yourself into alignment with your choice. It's a feeling game. And the good news is words have vibration and carry with them the vibrational imprint to help you align to it. If you say the word love out loud, you can actually feel its vibration in your body.

Try it now. Say aloud love. Say it over and over again. What do you feel? Be curious. Try this with other words such as anger, boredom, positive expectation, joy and peace.

You can't say I choose abundance and spend the rest of your day thinking thoughts of lack and vibrating in scarcity mulling over what you don't have. Nope. You must choose thoughts of abundance, feel yourself vibrating as abundance, and be in alignment with abundance for it to manifest in your life.

Self-awareness is key in evaluating what you are in resonance with. Through self-awareness you can use words that trigger feelings to bring you into alignment with your desires.

When you don't choose your thoughts, the world reflects back to you what has been chosen for you based upon past experiences, cultural dogma or doctrine, and distorted programs handed down ancestrally through generations. You are a feather floating in the wind and wherever the wind blows you go, whether you want to go there or not.

When you choose your thoughts and come into alignment with those thoughts, you choose your reality and the world will reflect back to you all that you have chosen. You are empowered. You have mastered this thing called mind and the vehicle called physical form.

Find peace in the quiet space between thoughts. Then choose consciously in full awareness what comes forth from that space and know in truth the power that lies within you.

Note on Manifestation: Do not ask for abundance. Ask for what abundance will give you and align with that. For example, will abundance give you freedom? Expression? Experience? These things are easy to align to because we have all felt them at one time or another. Simply remember a time when you felt free; feel that feeling within your body and boom! You are aligned and, powerful creator that you are, you will magnetize that to you. Use your imagination when choosing thoughts you wish to align to. Feel the playfulness of the universe. Do not beg, plead, command, demand, or approach creation with entitlement. Those things do not work. Trust me. Manifestation is best done with the spirit of a child who wants nothing more than to laugh, imagine, and try different things with no objective other than play.

Emotional Hairballs and Embedded Patterns

Certain thought patterns can create energy formations that can get lodged within your body. The more you repeat a thought, the deeper that pattern gets lodged until it becomes a deeply rooted belief, emotional imprint or what I call an emotional hairball, or egoic structure that you think is you.

As a child if you were told repeatedly that what you did was not good enough, the thought pattern "not good enough" becomes an energy form that is lodged within you. When that one thought takes possession of the mind, it can take control and become your whole universe. We talk about these embedded patterns and emotional hairballs when we talk about emotions. For now, as you cultivate awareness, simply be aware that certain emotions may arise to be released from the physical body and it's okay. If the urge to cry arises, cry. You may find yourself crying and you have absolutely no idea why. This is a very good sign the embedded pattern is unraveling. Emotions just want to be felt and let go.

Letting emotions such as anger, fear, and sadness flow through you and out of you may seem scary at first, but when you succeed at it once, you gain confidence. You discover you won't die and it actually feels quite good to let your emotions come and go without a story attached to them. Some compare it to the feeling of poison leaving the body. The key words to pick up on here are to feel your emotions *without a story attached to them*. If you get triggered and find yourself reacting to or getting caught up in an emotion, like a dog chewing on a bone, you have been hooked by an emotion and there is a story attached to it. Cultivate awareness and it will raise you above the story, enabling you to watch the emotion move through you and out of you.

Realize that this emotional hairball is an energy form that originated as a thought and is truly no more than a repetitive thought pattern reinforcing and feeding the energy form. It's like an old record that keeps playing over and over and over in your head.

When an embedded thought pattern arises, bring your

awareness to it. Say, "Oh, there's that old thought pattern" and it will lose its power. It's just an old tape from the past and the past holds no power over the present.

Awareness and discernment are the swords that dissolve embedded thought patterns.

As you continue to swing your sword of awareness and discernment, and choose your thoughts consciously, embedded patterns will begin to vaporize. This takes time, dedication, and patience.

In the beginning stages of awakening, the ego will fight for its survival because it thinks your conscious awareness is its death. Because thoughts are the content and form the structure of the ego, the ego doesn't go down without a fight. Don't let this deter you. Reassure your ego that it doesn't die, it transforms. The ego can be devious and find many ways to get you to identify with thoughts to reinforce a false identity. Every time this happens, send it love and thank it for trying to keep you safe.

It may seem like you just busted open a bee's nest and thoughts are like bees swarming all around you! While this is uncomfortable, it is normal. If waking up was easy, everyone would be doing it. Most people prefer to stay unconscious and not go through the discomfort of mastering their mind and redirecting it to bring more of what they desire.

But here you are.

You have chosen not to be unconsciously run by the thought patterns and programming of your past and experience yourself as a conscious sovereign being. Congratulations!

This means you will likely face uncomfortable emotions, moments of frustration, overwhelm, and difficulty. But swinging the swords of awareness and discernment need not be difficult. It need not be a struggle. You can literally zap each thought easily and instantaneously simply by bringing it into the light of your awareness. For example, let's say an embedded thought pattern arises, you increase awareness and discern it to be baloney, so you flick it off your shoulder and it dissolves. Simple. Not easy at times, but simple. When egoic thoughts are exposed to the light of consciousness, they dissolve.

Continue to invite awareness into your life. Be attentive. Get more and more comfortable being the witnesser and the conscious chooser of thoughts. Practice directing your mind to bring you new information instead of repeating the same old crap. Enjoy being in the space of no thought. There is such contentment here for you to enjoy.

It's not work; its choice, awareness, and alignment. And a lot of letting go. A mantra I create for many of my clients is: I am safe. Let go. Trust. Allow. Just be.

Over time the thoughts that used to thrash you will die down and fade away, leaving you in a state of soft, joyful beingness. You will experience more moments of no thought. Presence will grow within you as you invite it in and you create opportunities to experience that which you are. Then the mind becomes a tool that is used to bring you new information from the catalog of the universe.

Did I mention the importance of cultivating awareness?

MEDITATION: Sit in an upright posture and cast your eyes down to the floor at a 45 degree angle. Be aware of your sense perceptions, be aware of your physical body, be aware of your inner body, the silence, the stillness around and within you. Become super alert, like someone came up behind you and scared you. Now just wait for a thought to arise. What comes? Ask the mind to bring you something better. What does it bring? There is nothing more for you to do than cultivate awareness and choose. If any inspired action arises, take action. Action taken from elevated levels of awareness will be of a higher quality and often have greater impact with less struggle.

Each time you let go of a thought that doesn't serve you, you remember something new about yourself. It's the remembering that needs integration. The more you catch yourself indulging in a negative thought or old story of limitation and acknowledge it and let it go, the quicker the integration of the truth.

LAURI-ISM: Remembering helps you to forgive your illusions and trust your divinity. Your self-delusions and things you were taught from the past cannot take the place of the truth.

The Entire Journey

Becoming aware of your thoughts and choosing them consciously typically happens in many phases and the phases are different for everyone. These phases are taken from my own experience and the experiences of those with whom I've worked. The phases are not linear and you may jump back and forth between them for a while until you anchor yourself in each new way of being. In general, coming home to oneself begins with releasing and letting go of what is not true, letting go of what you are not, followed by an integration period of acclimating to the truth of who and what you really are.

Awareness and The Shitstorm.

Phase one is the slow process of awakening, where you come to realize just because you have thoughts doesn't mean they are true. This is the most difficult phase because your thoughts are like unruly children who haven't been disciplined. Chaos and compulsion abound. You believe many thoughts that arise and get snagged by them often. You spend a lot of time in your head, not in your heart.

This phase is marked by feeling totally out of control and your thoughts are like a shitstorm on fire pelting you from all directions. Feeling out of control is very normal in the beginning phases.

The ego is very active in the beginning because it has run the show for most of your life and the last thing it wants to do is hand over the reins to you. We'll talk more about how to deal with the ego in chapters to come.

In this phase you wrangle with your thoughts and ego and they win most of the time. You go back and forth between struggling with them, resisting them, hating them, and having moments where you are able to let them go. You may even have moments of no thoughts that encourage you to keep going.

Letting Go

You are getting better at discerning thoughts and flicking the thoughts that do not serve you off your shoulder. You are experiencing moments of peace.

This phase is marked by the feeling that you are constantly letting go.

As you begin to disidentify from the ego and understand it is not you, nor are you the thoughts it brings to you, you slowly peel away the layers of which you are not and start the process of returning the ego back to the faculty it originated as. You work with the ego, thank it, love it, and it slowly adapts. Your heart slowly opens.

Struggle and chaos with ups and downs exist in this phase and you ride them like a roller coaster. You are more of a witnesser of thoughts and don't get triggered as often. You still get hooked by a thought and go down the rabbit hole, but once you realize you are hooked, you are back in awareness. You sense you are being asked to give things up but may cling to certain attachments anyway.

You may witness the thoughts arising and leaving your field of consciousness without buying into them or getting triggered by them. You let them go. You let them go. You let them go. And you let them go. This book offers many creative linear and non-linear ways of letting go.

Over time you are more diligent in witnessing your thoughts, and thoughts no longer have the same hold on you. As Thomas Jefferson once said, "Eternal vigilance is the price of liberty," and you are the vigilant aware gatekeeper of thoughts. They may float into your consciousness, but you pay them no mind. They seem to be finer in quality, less intense, and more in the background of your life. Every once in a while an old thought pattern may arise to beat you up, but you recover fast and know that it is just an old pattern running its course. You become more and more familiar with yourself as the observer of your thoughts. Life has more peaceful moments where you experience your inner beingness.

You may feel like you have some sense of control, not in your ability to control whether a thought arises, but in your ability to let the thought go and redirect your mind to bring you something better. You start to understand how thoughts work and your role in choosing them and aligning to them. You become self-aware and know that whatever comes into your field of awareness is a result of the vibration you are putting out. Sometimes you like what arises, and sometimes you have to smack yourself in the forehead and laugh because what you manifested is not what truly serves you.

Identity Crisis

This is marked by a collapse of all that you thought you were. A feeling of being lost. You go back and forth between "Am I a human in physical form, or am I this aware presence?" And what the heck is this thing called aware presence? Feelings of being lost, yet found, certain and uncertain, knowing, yet completely in the dark.

When people reach this phase I congratulate them and they look at me like I'm crazy. This is a milestone and a necessary step, because as long as you're holding onto a false identity, you can't experience what you truly are.

Otherworldly experiences become more and more frequent and you go back and forth between, "Was that real or just my imagination?" Am I going crazy? is a common thought that arises.

Spiritual Significance

Extraordinary experiences of yourself become more comfortable and you gain confidence as you explore your multidimensionality. This is when spiritual significance can creep in, so be extra vigilant that the ego doesn't grab onto a new identity as spiritually advanced or superior. "I need to save the world, I am more advanced than you, or I have this huge responsibility" are identities the ego grabs onto. This is where a good integration guide can give you a universal bitch-slap and tell you to get off your high horse and get with the program. Tough love is needed to guide you away from both the feelings of lack of worthiness and the I am better than you complex. Remember, we are ALL Spirit in form; it's the new normal.

Super Awareness

This is when the thoughts get even finer and recede into the background of your life. You really have to pay close attention at this point as thoughts can slip by unnoticed. You continue to become more and more present with every now-moment, more and more aware of what you really are as Spirit in form and you continue to give up old behavior patterns that no longer serve you.

You start to understand your creator abilities and how powerful you are and you take responsibility for your creations. You become more aware of yourself as the presence that directs the faculty of the mind. You are getting better and better at saying, "Nope. That doesn't serve me. What else do you have?" and experience more moments of no thought.

It is not uncommon to experience moments of self-trust, self-love, joy, utter fulfillment, and euphoria. You may bounce back and forth between exquisite highs and lows of uncertainty and self-doubt. This is normal.

You are more and more curious about this thing called consciousness. You experience moments of self-compassion and love for the personality structure or persona called you.

Random thoughts that arise within your awareness give way to presence. Being. Peace. Simple being. No should/shouldn'ts, needs tos/have tos, cans/cannots, rights/wrongs, or good and bad. It's not that you don't take action, you do. The action arises from inspiration, not compulsion or reaction. Instead of judging others you may be tickled when you see other people and their creations. You get glimpses of who other people are beyond any story they have about themselves or any story you have about them. You start to release the illusion of control and fear. It doesn't happen all at once; it is a process that unfolds from moment to moment.

True Self Integration

The mind and you become a team. Your true nature becomes apparent. You clearly know you are a divine articulation that chooses freely what to do with any thought, situation, or experience that arises within your field of awareness.

You transition to being even more present, in peace, and in the beautiful now-moment. As you come into alignment with true self, distortions drop away. The choices you make are no longer in conflict because there is little to no doubt. It's like your white knuckles come off the wheel and you give up control and trust in this thing called being...but grab the wheel every once in a while just in case! You marvel at the mystery that bridges the gap between the divine and the physical. You trust that all is well, all unfolds.

The mind, now more connected to true self, may bring you information directing you or nudging you to go to a coffee shop, take a walk, cook some dinner, say hello to a stranger. You may find yourself in a grocery store not needing anything wondering why you are there, then meeting someone to offer a smile or a message.

You begin to engage more and more with whatever arises or

comes into your world from a place of choice. You know whatever comes into your field of awareness is a result of the vibration you are putting out and choose your thoughts consciously. You know you are the magnet that is attracting what comes to you. It is as if God is now before you with a silver platter saying, "How about this? Would you like to choose this?" And you may choose with the glee of a child whatever you like from that silver plate. It is a gift. You know you are in a constant state of receiving. You are no longer resisting. And your life and what you receive delights and surprises you. You understand why all ascended masters laugh so much.

You are not being bombarded by this false or separate entity called the ego. The ego becomes a divine faculty of love that acts as a bridge between you and the divine enabling you to receive and experience all the information in the universe.

Your soul, in a sense, descends and integrates within physicality. You experience Oneness, one with All That Is...yet remain an individual expression of the One and you know who and what you are without a doubt. You reside more and more in a place of no thought. You leave time and space and in many ways are no longer a human. The quality of your expressions and creations is much greater than ever before.

You understand that there is nothing you have to do, need to do, or should do. The ideas of right or wrong or good or bad disappear and you replace them with choice and experience for the sake of experience. You no longer feel you have to save the world or do things because you feel they make you a good person. You know your value is in your being. The mind becomes a tool, a faculty that can be used for logistics to be able to function in time and space to communicate and share.

The persona is no longer split; there is no longer an ego or small self and you as the observer or true self. There is a melding, a returning of the ego to the faculty and the personality or identity self disappears. There is no identity. You reside in being. That which you are cannot be described, contained, known, or limited by any idea of what it is.

These, of course, are just signposts that lead the way based upon my own experience and the experience of others. Many more levels are in between and beyond that are subtle and experiential, and it is not unusual to bounce around from one phase to the other and back again as you integrate and adapt to the information coming to you in each phase. In general though, the level of chaos and compulsion die down to be replaced with beingness, lightheartedness, ease, and a lovely, soft, joyful glow.

Certain thoughts that trigger lower vibrational frequency experiences, such as judgment, fear, anxiety, worry, guilt, and shame, arise and fall throughout all phases. Again, this is not a linear process.

INTEGRATE: Stop here and integrate this information. Ponder it. Where are you in the process of mastering your mind? While reading this section, what emotions arise within you? Are you excited? Or have you created a story that you have a long way to go?

How is your mind or ego reacting to this information? Be curious. Can you let go of any story and allow yourself to be where you are without judgment or significance?

Set aside some time now and create Truth Cards. My friend Aydika James came up with the idea of Truth Cards and they have helped many people come into alignment with their truths.

To create a Truth Card, place a piece of information that resonates with you onto an index card. Be sure to choose the words carefully so they create a positive vibrational frequency in your body when you read them. Be positive. For instance, don't write down "I am not unworthy." The word unworthy carries with it a code or frequency. It is much better to write down, "I am worthy."

For example, you could create cards that remind you of the main topics of this chapter. Such as:

- I am an articulation of the divine, spirit in physical form.

- The ego is a faculty of the mind that brings me information in the form of thoughts.

- I am the aware presence, the discerner of my thoughts.

- I am the chooser of my thoughts, the director of my mind.

- Through awareness I know when I am in alignment with my choice

- I know I am aligned by how I feel. I feel good when I am aligned with truth.

Or you could create Truth Cards that give you a sense of relief as you let go of the old and adapt to the new. Such as:

- I am safe

- I am free

- Let go

- Trust

- Open

- Receive

Choose anything from this book, another book, a meditation, or information revealed to you in a plant medicine journey. Choose things you want to remember and embody. Here are a few powerful ones that have really helped me:

- I don't need to know

- Peace

- Just be

- Love

These cards carry the vibrational frequency of what is written on them and will help activate, integrate, and anchor the energy and truth within you. Use colored pens or pencils, get artistic with watercolors if you like, and doodle. The more energy and creativity you put into remembering, integrating, and applying this information, the more it will become a part of your life. Leave them laying around your house as reminders.

If Truth Cards don't resonate and you like to journal, scan back through the chapter and write in your journal the important points you would like to integrate. Go through the information in these chapters until you feel complete with the content before moving on.

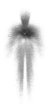

CHAPTER 4:

BELIEFS, PART ONE

Quick Recap: In the last chapter you discovered that thoughts and words have vibrational frequencies you experience in the body and that you create via thoughts by utilizing choice, self-awareness, and vibrational alignment. You found that certain thought patterns can create energy formations that can get lodged within your body called emotional imprints or hairballs. Awareness is the sword that dissolves negative thought patterns and can cause these hairballs to surface in order to be released and let go. You learned a meditation that will assist you in retraining the mind to bring you better information and you read how your entire journey to awaken may unfold. If something is unclear, ask your mind to fetch you clarity and create the space to receive what it brings you. It is quite extraordinary when the mind is properly utilized and directed.

Now let's delve into beliefs.

What Are Beliefs?

When you think the same thing over and over again it becomes a repetitive energy pattern in your mind and body and becomes a belief. That's what a belief is: it's a thought that's been thought over and over and over again. Because of the repetition, beliefs can become deeply rooted into our biology. The more we think something the deeper it burrows into the body-mind and the tougher it can be to dislodge.

So it makes sense that if 80 percent of the thoughts you have each day are negative and false, then the majority of your beliefs must also be negative and false. Wow! Sit with that for a moment. 80 percent. Negative. False.

Beliefs, just like thoughts, are unreliable. Just because you hold a belief, doesn't mean it's true.

Inherited Beliefs

The scientific community is giving more and more credence to the role our beliefs play in determining our physiologies and our realities. And there are many types of beliefs, but none so easily embedded as those that are given to us by the people around us. For example, a parent may believe his child is incapable and unknowingly pass this belief onto the child. A parent may pass on a work ethic or an ancestral pattern of physical or mental abuse or trauma. Grandparents may have believed that another ethnic group is inferior and passed that belief down.

Many people inherit the patterns of fear, self-doubt, depression, hopelessness, worry, and anxiety from their parents, who inherited it from their parents, who inherited it from their parents and so on. Inherited beliefs can come from the collective, such as shared ideas and moral attitudes, which often operate as a unifying force within society that become rules and laws, regardless of the validity of the beliefs.

What beliefs have you inherited from your parents or from the world around you?

REFLECTIVE MOMENT: Patterns of depression, hopelessness, worry, and anxiety are projections of what might happen in the future with the attachment of a story. They are not real. These are often patterns that we learned from our parents or the world around us. The things we worry about rarely or never happen. If you experience these feelings on a regular basis, ponder them. Did you inherit them? If you were taught how to feel this way by your parents or others, can you learn a new way? You don't have to let them go; you can hold on to them if you wish, just consider what your life would be like without them.

Your Life Reflects Your Beliefs

Regardless of whether a belief is true or not, your life reflects that belief. What you believe shows up in your life in observable ways. Now stay with me here; this is some big stuff. If you look at your life openly and curiously you will see that your life is a reflection of your belief system. This can be hard for some people to hear, especially if they don't like the way their life is going. You can affirm this by looking at your life. Every day, you act out your belief system in the things you do, the things you say, and the actions you take. For instance:

• If you work 60 hours each week, you believe that work is more important than other things. Your life reflects that belief, whether the belief is conscious or unconscious.

• If you believe you don't have time to eat well and take care of yourself, I don't have time is a belief that unfolds in your life.

• If you don't believe exercise is important, you may not do it.

• If you don't believe you are worth taking care of, you may take care of everyone but yourself.

Your beliefs show up in how you prioritize your day and by what is important to you.

Look at your daily routine. From the time you get up to the time you go to bed, where do you spend the most time?

1 a.m.

2 a.m.

3 a.m.

4 a.m.

5 a.m.

6 a.m.

7 a.m.

8 a.m.

9 a.m.

10 a.m.

11 a.m.

12 p.m.

1 p.m.

2 p.m.

3 p.m.

4 p.m.

5 p.m.

6 p.m.

7 p.m.

8 p.m.

9 p.m.

10 p.m.

11 p.m.

12 a.m.

REFLECTIVE MOMENT: How did you fill out the timeline above? Where do you spend most of your time? What are you doing for the majority of your day? Are your actions congruent with what you truly believe to be important in your life?

Beliefs do change. For example, your partner may have different political beliefs than you, but as the relationship evolves you or your partner may shift political beliefs so you are in alignment. Or you may think something is silly or a waste of time, even though you have never tried it. Once you do try it and have a better understanding of it, you may change your mind about its value or how fun it is.

Often once people see how silly an old belief really is they can let it go quite easily. Just seeing it in truth dissolves it.

If you were to shift your daily activities to reflect what you consciously and truly believe is most important to you, how would your daily routine unfold? What would your day look like?

1 a.m.

2 a.m.

3 a.m.

4 a.m.

5 a.m.

6 a.m.

7 a.m.

8 a.m.

9 a.m.

10 a.m.

11 a.m.

12 p.m.

1 p.m.

2 p.m.

3 p.m.

4 p.m.

5 p.m.

6 p.m.

7 p.m.

8 p.m.

9 p.m.

10 p.m.

11 p.m.

12 a.m.

Is this something you can gift yourself? Even if you can't make all the changes you desire right away, what little things can you let go of or bring into your day to come into alignment with your beliefs?

Beliefs Around Yourself

- If you believe yourself to be unworthy, your experience of yourself will reflect that belief, whether the belief is conscious or unconscious.

- If you believe you aren't smart enough, pretty enough, or confident enough, your experience of yourself will reflect that belief.

- If you believe you're a failure, that will be your reality.

• If you believe you are less than others, that will be your experience.

• If you believe you have to behave a certain way to be loved, that will manifest in your relationships.

• If you believe this physical body is all you are that will be your experience.

On the flip side:

• If you believe yourself to be worthy, you will feel and be valued and loved.

• If you believe you're smart, beautiful, and confident, your experience of yourself will reflect that belief.

• If you believe you're a success, that will be your experience.

• If you believe love is unconditional, that will manifest as your experience.

• If you believe you are spirit riding this crazy thing called a body for the experience of it, that will be how you live here on earth.

Your beliefs become a self-fulfilling prophecy.

Both so-called positive identities and negative identities arise from beliefs, and beliefs are used to create false identities. For example, depending on your beliefs, you may view a politician as a "world changer" or as "an evil person," and in reality, the person is neither.

Or you can see a person who lives in a nice, maybe enviable home, and give them the label "successful" when that person may see themselves as "unsuccessful" because they are actually heavily in debt. And the final example is someone who has been abused, could create the identity of being a survivor (positive identity) or a victim (negative identity).

All identities––positive or negative—are false as they are stories we tell ourselves and the meanings we attach are arbitrary. There is no truth in any of these beliefs. They are judgments of right and wrong, good and bad, should and shouldn'ts—social constructs we have agreed to in some way or another that do nothing but pigeonhole us and put us in boxes.

All beliefs are limitations. All beliefs are used to create false identities.

You are not just a doctor, a politician, a social worker, or a grocery checker. You are not just a mom, a dad, a brother or sister; you are not just an artist or an engineer. You are not the things you do, the money you make, the house you live in, or the car you drive. You are none of these things.

> **MEDITATION:** What false identities have you created? Sit with an erect posture and be perfectly still. Be aware of your body and where it is located in the room and any sounds that arise in stillness without judgment. Now strip away your name, the work you do, the roles you play and any beliefs you have about yourself.

What do you discover about yourself? Can you feel it? Strip away all that you are not, and for a moment, experience what is.

Beliefs Around Money

Your relationship with money will also give you insights into your beliefs.

- If you believe money is bad, you likely won't have much of it.

- If you believe money makes you a bad person you may avoid it.

- If you believe money can contribute to the betterment of the world, you most likely use money to do just that.

- If you believe you have to work hard and struggle to make money that will most likely be your experience.

- If money comes to you quickly and easily with great joy, you most likely hold the belief that that's what money does.

- If you believe your services are only worth so much, you may set your rates low so your receivership matches your belief.

REFLECTIVE MOMENT: What if you had the belief that money was the degree in which you allow yourself to be loved by the universe? How would your relationship with money change? If you removed all threads of good/bad, right/wrong, need to/have to, should/shouldn't from money and any story of how you have to sacrifice or work hard to get it, what would you experience?

Conflicting Beliefs

Some people have conflicting beliefs regarding money and a whole range of subjects. Conflicting beliefs are the ones that really throw the universe for a loop and explain while we may not be manifesting our desires effectively. For instance:

• You may believe that certain foods are bad for you, and you must give them up to lose weight. But on the other hand, you love those foods and can't imagine life without them. You are in conflict.

• You may believe you need money to be fulfilled in life. But you believe money is bad. You are in conflict.

• You may believe you need a relationship to fulfill you, yet believe you are unworthy of the relationship. Conflict.

• You may believe that you are an aspect of the divine, but don't believe yourself to be worthy of that gift. Conflict.

• You may believe you need to quit your job to be happy, yet believe you can't quit your job because you need the money. More conflict.

Is it any wonder we manifest anything? No wonder the universe brings us a mixed bag of what we desire. What we send out is a mixed bag of requests.

REFLECTIVE MOMENT: Look at the conflicts below.

Not worthy of love...need it to be fulfilled
Not worthy of money...need it to be fulfilled
Not worthy of success...need it to be fulfilled
Not worthy of happiness...need it to be fulfilled
Not worthy of losing weight...need it to be fulfilled

What else might you feel that you are not worthy of, yet feel like you need it to be fulfilled? Do you see where so many of us get stuck?

Seeing the conflict helps to unravel it because we see the madness. When you strip anything of meaning, it just becomes, "What do you want?" Then you are free to go after what tickles your fancy. Not because it will make you a better person, more spiritual, or enhance your identity, but because it is something you choose simply because you want to.

INTEGRATION: All beliefs are limitations. All beliefs are used to create false identities. There is no such thing as identity. All identities are false. You are not the roles you play; you are not the stuff you have. There is no such thing as worthiness. No good/bad, right/wrong, or judgment of any kind. Sit with this information. Be with it. Explore it, question it, and find out if it's true for you before you move on to the next chapter.

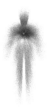

CHAPTER 5:

BELIEFS, PART TWO

Quick Recap: In the previous chapter you learned that when you think the same thing over and over again it becomes a repetitive energy pattern in the body mind and becomes a belief structure. If 80% of the thoughts you have each day are negative and false, then the majority of your beliefs must also be negative and false. You explored beliefs inherited from your parents and the world around you and saw how your life reflects your beliefs and beliefs can change. You had many reflective moments while you explored your own beliefs and where they may be in conflict. You learned all beliefs are limitations, and beliefs are used to create false identities. You are not the roles you play; you are not the stuff you have. There is no such thing as worthiness. You are free to choose and create whatever you desire just because you can. Isn't that a relief? You did a meditation designed to strip you of what you are not in order to experience that which you are. How did that go?

Now, let's continue our exploration of beliefs.

Beliefs Around Food

This is one area where people get stuck A LOT. Our relationship with food is another example that will give us many insights into our beliefs about ourselves. For instance,

- If you believe certain foods are bad for you, when you eat those foods you may experience guilt and shame. Those foods may also impact your body in so-called "bad" ways and you may feel awful when you eat them.

- You may believe you need to lose weight to be fulfilled, and in order to do that, you believe you should starve yourself. But on the other hand, you are a human being who eats! Big conflict.

- If you believe all food is meant to be enjoyed and savored, you may have a love relationship with your food.

- If you believe all food nourishes you, all foods may nourish your body deeply and you may feel great when you eat them.

- If you don't believe eating fruits and vegetables is

delicious, they likely won't be.

- If you believe you have to eat protein with every meal, you may experience anxiety when you don't.

You may believe you need to avoid certain foods to be healthy, yet you love those foods. Big conflict.

If you believe that you are not worthy of love or good things in your life, that you are not allowed to have what you want, or that there is not enough, those feelings may show up in your relationship with food and you may binge trying to get enough or to be enough.

Looking at our world today and all the crazy belief structures it makes sense that so many of us are miserable! Remember 80 percent of the thoughts we think each day are negative and false! And 95 percent of those are repetitive.

Again, regardless of whether they are true or not, our beliefs create our lives and realities.

Storytime: Consider this: Alia Crum, a clinical psychologist, did a study where she gave a group of people a 380-calorie milkshake under the pretense that it was either a 620-calorie "indulgent" shake or a 140-calorie "sensible" shake. She then measured the levels of ghrelin. Ghrelin is a hormone that increases when we are hungry, which drives us to go hunt and gather food. When we find food, ghrelin increases metabolism to digest and absorb what we have eaten. It also slows metabolism in the case that we don't find food.

In the study, participants were asked to rate the milkshake, and ghrelin levels were measured. After individuals consumed the "indulgence" shake, they reported feeling very satisfied with the experience, and their levels of ghrelin decreased dramatically, and their metabolisms kicked in to begin digesting and utilizing the nutrients. Then, when individuals consumed the "sensible" shake, it produced a relatively flat ghrelin response. They reported not feeling as satisfied, and metabolism was not triggered to the same degree. And it was the exact same milkshake for both groups!

In short, the degree in which their metabolism kicked in was consistent with what they *believed* they were drinking. Not the actual nutritional value of the shake.

This explains why one person can eat bacon cheeseburgers regularly without gaining weight, and another person just has to take one bite and gains ten pounds! Living a healthy life is not only about managing your food intake; it is also about managing your thoughts, beliefs, and emotions.

Dissolving embedded belief structures and changing your perspective will help you not only shift your biology, but also can change your life and your reality.

REFLECTIVE MOMENT: What do you think would happen if you stopped judging food, put away the guilt and shame, and instead of listening to what everyone else says you should or shouldn't eat, you tuned into your body? If you ate when your body was hungry, and stopped when it was satisfied, and paid attention to its responses to the food you gave it, what would you learn?

My Relationship with Food

When I discovered that everything I was taught about food, alcohol, and coffee was relative to my beliefs about it and my mentor told me not to judge what I chose, I was paralyzed!

I had spent my whole life eating what everyone else told me I should eat and I had no idea how my body actually responded to food. Really? I could have alcohol and not be a bad person or gain weight? Really? I could eat whatever I wanted? My beliefs around food were the hardest for me to unwind. No matter how many times Lauri told me not to judge what I ate, I couldn't help it.

When I went through school to become a nutrition professional I had been taught the good food-bad food paradigm and honestly believed that food was my enemy. If I didn't eat a perfect diet, I was off the wagon beating myself over the head with guilt and shame. The paradigm at that time was legumes and rice contained carbs, toxins, and arsenic. Coffee, alcohol, sugar, fast food, junk food, processed foods, tilapia, and other farm-raised fish were also bad. We were told to avoid fruits because they are high in sugar, certain vegetables because of genetic modification and pesticides, and certain animal proteins because of growth hormones. Honestly, eating according to all the rules made me crazy. It's no wonder so many of us look at food as the enemy. But it's not the enemy, it's our beliefs about food that is the enemy.

This took me a long time to understand, so I will say this again in a different way. Food in itself is not good or bad; it's what you believe about it that makes it good or bad. Remember, you are a powerful creator and you create with your thoughts and beliefs. If you come into alignment with the belief that eating certain foods or drinking is bad, then you are aligning to a construct that will trigger guilt and shame when you indulge in those things. You are not creating a construct where you are aligning with freedom of choice.

Instead, look at food as cause and effect. And cause and effect isn't doctrine, it's how that food affects *your* body when you eat it. Cause and effect most importantly takes into consideration your beliefs and vibrational alignment with those beliefs. For example, if you set the belief that you and your body have a love affair with food and your body delights and can handle whatever you choose, and then you eat ice cream and experience an underlying feeling of guilt, you are not in alignment. Your body is different from everyone else's. No one else can tell you how your body does with foods or whether you are in alignment with your beliefs. Only you know.

As I explored my beliefs around food I found intuitive eating to be helpful because it forced me to go within and rely on the wisdom of my body. Instead of relying on a belief or construct that was outside of me, I relied on my inner wisdom. Then I came up against the real problem. The problem wasn't that I was eating the right/wrong foods. My body actually did very well with bacon cheeseburgers and French fries. The problem was I would check in with my body and it would call for vegetables and for a few days I would honor that. But then as I started feeling good my mind would sabotage me and I'd end up going through the McDonalds drive-thru. Guilt and shame and the old belief pattern of self-judgment resurfaced. I knew what I wanted to do; I just couldn't seem to do it. Why couldn't I listen to my body? Why was my mind always sabotaging me?

Then I realized that my entire belief system about myself was based on myself as unworthy. I believed that it was not okay to shine or step into my power. And as soon as I started to move outside of the construct of unworthiness, the belief that it was not okay to shine pulled me back in. I was being controlled subconsciously by an old belief that no longer served me. On top of it all, when I faced this and brought it to the surface I was afraid. I was really afraid of who I would be if I took care of myself, loved myself, and was healthy. I had an identity crisis. I used to say that good nutrition practitioners implore people to make changes. Great practitioners empower their clients to feel safe to make a transition of identity.

LAURI-ISM: Food is an empowerment of choice and a freedom of choice, rather than a need of a substance.

Now there are many layers to my predicament: there was a false identity I had created as unworthy, the belief I had created that someone who shines is bad, the construct of good foods and bad foods and what it meant if I chose those foods. Then there was the issue of safety. I did not feel safe to move into a new construct or identity.

It's true that the one thing we fear the most is that we are more powerful than we ever imagined ourselves to be. Yup. I'd taste a bit of that power and shrink back from it by taking a deep dive into food and alcohol to feel safe. I wasn't choosing food freely;

I *needed* it to feed, soothe, and avoid my emotions.

In order for me to leave the old construct of an unworthy, stuck being and become a free and conscious chooser, I had to face the discomfort of feeling good. I know that sounds insane, but it is true. I had to shine the light of awareness on the old construct, face the discomfort of not residing in that construct any longer, and get used to feeling good.

Was it uncomfortable? Definitely. Did I falter? I can't count the times my body asked for a light meal and I binged on way too much food. I faltered many times. I approached my new identity slowly and acclimated to the idea a little at a time. I struggled and overcame and struggled and adapted. Is it worth the struggle? Absolutely. The cravings, the addiction to self-deprecation, the fear, the shrinking, the chaos, and the compulsion and the feeling of lack, these are worth moving beyond. Today I know there are things that I choose that will evolve me, and there are things I do, that will not evolve me. There is no judgment if I choose an old pattern, but I know there is freedom and expansion when I move beyond it.

To reiterate, it was my awareness of the beliefs and identity construct that dissolved the discomfort of feeling good. It was my willingness to transition to a new identity that bridged the gap. It didn't happen overnight, and to be honest, I still have moments where it flashes before my eyes. But the difference now is I see the beliefs come and go instead of getting triggered or being driven by them. I see the old identity and lift my chin in gratitude for where I am.

When it comes to your relationship with food and yourself I

recommend practicing compassion. Accept what is and where you are knowing you will soon move out of the uncomfortable phase of letting go and acclimate to the truth of yourself. Compassion is the ticket that leads to self-trust, patience, empowerment of choice, and eventually, self-love.

> **REFLECTIVE MOMENT:** What beliefs, identity constructs, or patterns do you hold around food or yourself that could be dissolved with your conscious awareness? What identity transition would you like to make?

We will talk more about how to handle emotions that may arise when you consider a transition of identity in the chapters to come. For now, know that any fear that arises is false. Fear is a projection of a future event with the attachment of a story. Remove the story and just allow yourself to be.

In truth, the process of evolution is exchanging one limiting belief for a less limiting belief until you realize all beliefs are limitations. It's exchanging one identity for another until you realize all identities are limitations. This is when you come home to yourself as an unlimited being exploring limitations for the sake of experience. You then, as my friend Lauri likes to say, "Wear the costume loosely."

Today I continue to peel away the constructs of identity and the collective constructs around food and alcohol. I love a good bourbon and an occasional cigar. I love getting together with my sister and good friends for our yearly camping trip where we hike, raft, drink, and smoke cigarettes while I lose money at cards. I love a wonderful, well prepared meal. I am moving toward a mostly vegetarian diet but still choose a good steak or salted, roasted chicken from time to time.

I have found that it is more important to choose what I do based on my own preferences. I am not judged if I choose to eat conventional meat, but it feels better to me to consume animal proteins who have been raised with love and treated humanely. I appreciate organic fruits and vegetables grown without modification or pesticides because that's what resonates with me. But I am not sent to a fiery hell if I choose a big juicy conventional apple. Nor is anyone else.

I am now very aware when addiction comes calling. When freedom of choice gives way to a feeling of need...or I have to. This goes for my addiction to certain thought patterns and belief structures. Tobacco has, in fact, been one of my greatest teachers and I will never again consider it "bad."

LAURI-ISM: Your relationship with truth is whatever you subjugate it to. If you're not happy with your day when you lay your head on the pillow at night that's your dysfunction with you.

I am very alert for when I might be out of balance. I'm aware of whether I have freedom of choice because I simply want to, or if I'm getting pulled into an addictive cycle of needing to feed, soothe, or avoid something.

107

You truly do get to choose. The question is, are you choosing unconsciously and being driven by the chaos and compulsion of social constructs, negative thoughts, limiting beliefs, and false identities? Or are you choosing consciously as a sovereign awake and aware divine being?

MEDITATION: Cultivate awareness as you go about your day. Is there any time you feel you *need* something in order to avoid discomfort? Do you *need* to watch TV? Do you *need* to have that drink? Do you *need* to eat when you aren't hungry? Are you using these things to avoid your emotions or to avoid being present with yourself? If so, just stop for a moment and spend two minutes with your eyes closed, breathing deeply, and relaxing. Watch the discomfort fade. Then ask yourself, "What is it I really desire? What is it that I really hunger for in life?" Then choose from a place of awareness.

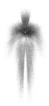

CHAPTER 6:

BELIEFS, PART THREE

Quick Recap: In the last chapter we explored our beliefs about food and how the degree in which our body responds to food is consistent with what we believe about that food. Not the actual nutritional value. You had more moments of reflection on what would happen if you stopped judging food, put away the guilt and shame, and instead of listening to what everyone else says you tuned into your body. You learned how to eat intuitively. You learned how to discern between choosing something simply because you want to, and being compulsively pulled into an addictive cycle of needing to. You did a meditation to help you discover what you really hunger for in life. What did you discover?

Let us continue on with beliefs.

Questioning Your Beliefs

Most people don't question their beliefs. When you are curious about your beliefs and are honest, open, and truthful about them, that's when you have the power to change them.

Many people say, "I don't have time to meditate," "I don't have time to cook," "I don't have time to exercise," or "I don't have time to do this workbook." I don't have time is a belief that shows up throughout their lives. They are living to reach some far-off goal that never arrives. To this, I respond, "You do have time. You just have the limiting belief that you don't."

The problem isn't that you don't have time. The problem is you believe that you don't have time. To solve this problem, you break down this limiting belief and *voila*, you have time!

When you dissect the belief "I don't have time," you see there's always a way to make things work; sometimes you just need to inquire as to whether your beliefs are serving you.

Being without negative thoughts and limiting belief patterns is freeing. It's calm, peaceful, and laced with a deep contentment that is delicious!

Often we fear losing our identity when we release repetitive thoughts and limiting beliefs with which we identify, and to some degree this is very accurate. We do lose identity, false identity.

LAURI-ISM: Dissolving each repetitive thought pattern, each energetic belief structure is like taking off a hat that represents a false identity. As you do this, you will find yourself taking off hat after hat after hat. The ego will fight a bit and put a hat back on, but if you are tenacious and dedicated, eventually that hat comes off and you finally get to discover the truth of who you are beneath all the hats.

The Six Phases of Change

When you question beliefs the mind can be very stubborn. Most people can relate to the statement, "I know what I need to do, I just can't seem to do it." So it often helps to have mind hacks. This next section shares an excellent way to trick the mind into letting go of a belief.

Any time you are thinking about taking off a hat or releasing any belief, the mind quickly goes to work to determine if the change will be beneficial. It evaluates the consequences of this new change to yourself and others. This is often done unconsciously. If the mind determines the change not to be beneficial or experiences inner conflict, the change is less likely to occur.

The book, *Changing for Good*, was written by three psychologists, James O. Prochaska, John Norcross, and Carlo DiClemente, who spent much of their lives studying the nature of change. They found that people generally move through six phases when trying to overcome embedded beliefs, habits, and patterns.

1. Pre-contemplation: You aren't even thinking about change.
2. Contemplation: You are contemplating making a change.
3. Preparation: You prepare to make a change.
4. Action: You are in action taking the steps to make change happen.
5. Maintenance: You continue to take action until it becomes a part of you and second nature. You have new embedded patterns.
6. Completion: You don't even think about it anymore. It is second nature.

This is really important: When your mind analyzes the pros and cons of making any change, if your list of cons is more emotionally charged and longer than your pros, change can be difficult because your mind is not on board. Your mind perceives the change as not being worthwhile. You have inner conflict. You have to get your mind's buy-in in order for you to perceive the change as worth it.

You have to dissolve the repetitive thoughts and embedded beliefs so the mind will get on board. Of course this is done with awareness.

I did mention the importance of cultivating awareness, did I not?

Sorry, I digress. Again, the mind must perceive more pros than cons and the pros must be more emotionally compelling than the cons for the mind to buy into the change.

EXERCISE: Think about a behavior you would like to change. Then use the chart below (or create a pro and con column on a piece of paper or in your journal). Let your mind go free and write down the pros and cons about changing this behavior. Don't censor anything. Get petty and write whatever comes to mind no matter how silly.

Pros	Cons

When you are done, look at your columns. Is your pro column longer or shorter than the con column? Which one is more emotionally charged?

Changing Your Perceptions

Now what we are going to do is change your perceptions. This is a fun, mind-bending exercise that exemplifies our ability to change our reality simply by changing our thoughts and beliefs.

1. Do The Work: Go back to your CONS lists and use Byron Katie's four questions; do The Work on each statement and draw a line through any con that is not true.

1. Is it true?
2. Can you absolutely know that it's true?
3. How do you react, what happens, when you believe that thought?
4. Who would you be without the thought?

Then turn the thought around. For example, "It's hard" becomes "it's not hard or it's easy." "I don't have time" becomes "I do have time." Think in terms of opposites.

*Don't skip a step. This must be experiential. FEEL your way through each con so the truth of it lands as a knowing. Be willing to just hang with and trust the answers that come. Trust the truth will be revealed.

2. Emotionally Charge Your Pros: Now look at your PROS lists and see if you have any additional pros to add. The goal is to have twice as many pros and have them be more emotionally charged.

When you read your pros column, it should really excite you. When you look at your con column, it shouldn't give you reason to pause. This exercise allows the inner conflict to be resolved in your subconscious mind, so that you can make the changes you want without hesitation.

What can you add to your pro column?

Now, be sure your pro list is longer by 50 percent and more emotionally compelling.

Congratulations! You just changed perspectives and shifted your beliefs! Changing your perspective can resolve inner conflict and change your habits and reality. Every behavior has a positive intention. For example to bring us love, safety, or belonging. Changing the beliefs, changes the identity, and changes the behavior.

The more you shine the light of awareness onto negative thoughts and limiting beliefs the less frequently they will arise and make their way out of the body. It just takes consistency and dedication. It is a choice.

You are responsible for your beliefs. The comfort zone is a prison. Being uncomfortable is where growth and fulfillment can be found. Being willing is half the battle. Once you use awareness to dissolve a negative thought or a limiting belief it gets easier and easier. It just takes time and repetition.

Beliefs Are Constructs

Beliefs are all constructs, and all constructs are limitations. The world we live in today is composed of construct after construct after construct. Everything we just talked about, your life, yourself, the money you earn, your beliefs about food are all constructs. Collective agreements that we think are fact, but they are not. They are subjective agreements based on past information that become doctrine.

LAURI-ISM: You are given a gift of presence, given your own pen to write your own story. You can go into the mystery or repeat the same old story. It's up to you. You can take from the constructs what you like or leave them altogether.

The choices you have before you are based on one thing and one thing only: God gave you the gift of life. He said, "Here is a world, do as you will!" and we've all got our panties in a stitch because we think we *should* be doing this and we *should* be doing that. When we buy into these religious doctrines or governmental decrees, we miss out on what we really would love to be doing.

Strike the words should/shouldn't, right/wrong, good/bad, need to/have to, or must do from your vocabulary and replace them with I choose to. And if you didn't consciously choose something in your life that is making you miserable, drop it! If you can't drop it, at least come up with a plan to work towards what you want.

In one of my meditations I kept repeating, right/wrong,

good/bad, judgment... blech! It was like I was spitting out the constructs and distortions we've all been caught in. I saw the entire VR room as one big construct and like all constructs... it changes.

A small-scale example of this is the construct that vegetable oil was healthy. In the 1950s we moved away from animal fats and butter to vegetable oil because it was promoted and advertised as healthier and saturated fats got the label "bad." Beliefs changed. The constructs around animal fats changed. Then recently the beliefs around vegetable oil changed again and the new construct became "vegetable oil is hydrogenated and therefore no longer healthy." Now some people believe vegetable oil to be healthy and some believe animal fats to be the healthier choice. Which is true? *Whichever you believe it to be.* Both are beliefs; both are constructs. Both are limitations.

Now just hang in here with me for a bit; this is some big stuff.

On a larger scale look at the VR room. Look at what many call the Matrix. It is a construct. A construct in which many of the inhabitants agreed to come into physical form and forget who they are to answer the question, "Who am I?" Let's face it, what better way to know the self than to forget the self and rediscover it from a different perspective? The VR room here on Earth is a construct of forgetting to remember. Now it is evolving and becoming a construct in which its inhabitants know who they are and are free to create without the distortions that arose from forgetting.

Yes, our world is a construct. My point here is that all beliefs are limitations and that includes the beliefs you have about yourself. You, dear one, are free to choose whatever you like from the smorgasbord of life without any meaning attached to it whatsoever.

Life Beyond the Construct

When you see that all beliefs are limitations, you drop them one by one. You become a free sovereign being without need, without identity, without negative thoughts or belief patterns in your field of awareness, and life gets really fun. You stop reacting and start choosing. You may go back and forth for a while with your foot in and out of the construct until you realize that while you live within the construct, within the VR room, you are not of the VR room. You reside more and more in being that which you are. You start to see others for who they are beyond the stories they have about them and the constructs they have created.

The more you let go of negative thoughts and limiting beliefs, the more fun you have. You laugh at the ridiculousness of humanity and say, "Good on you!" knowing everyone has a right to their own creations, their own inner and outer worlds, and you start to see that everything is creation. A thought is a creation. A belief is a creation. An identity is a creation. You, dear one, are creation!

When I experienced myself outside of all constructs it was so overwhelmingly beautiful I fell to my knees and shook my head. And for the longest time I felt I had to be like Jesus or the Buddha...until I realized that they had created those identities and at the core of their existence, what resides within them also resides within me. Beyond the constructs of those identities we are the same. The same consciousness that is within them lies within all beings.

It took me a long time to give up the idea of piousness of who I *should* emulate, how I *should* act, or what I *should* do with my life. Now, do I absolutely love and adore those beings for their contribution to the world? Absolutely. Do I *need* to be like them to be good enough? No. There is only one me. No one else sees the world like I do. Am I inspired by their work? Absolutely. But I see their work wasn't a result of what they did, it was who and what they were. They walked divinity. They embodied it. This inspires me to align with new levels of awareness, new vibrational frequencies, and choose ever-expanding experiences of my true self. What will this look like? Who knows! Do I still fall on my face? Sure. But it certainly is exciting!

When making your own decisions, it may be helpful to consider the way in which you intend to be, the means by which you live by. That may be helpful in the daily choices you see before you. But don't do things because they will make you a good person. Choose them because you are inspired to. Because it is an expression that wants to be born through you.

So an awakening being can be a cigar smoking, bourbon drinking gal, a dope smoking housewife, a homeless man, an entrepreneur, or a scientist. The self-realizing human doesn't look a certain way. It doesn't look like Gandhi, Jesus, or any other ascended master, although if you want to emulate a master, fine. Just remember that there are no shoulds or shouldn'ts or rights or wrongs that you must adhere to. Enlightenment, dear one, is the new normal. You are extraordinarily ordinary, and we are all on the same path towards it.

I was driving home one day listening to AC/DC and the song *Let Me Put My Love Into You* came on. I had this vision of God expressing himself and singing to me as that human up on the stage rocking out and I was laughing through the whole song.

We are all divine beings in physical form for the experience of it, for the wisdom gained, to undergo losing ourselves and finding ourselves. There is no right or wrong or way that enlightenment should look like. The enlightened human is the new construct. It is the new normal and you and I, dear one, are leading the way.

A natural tendency on the path of enlightenment is to transition away from overconsumption and to have more concern for the welfare of all life on the planet. As a person matures, they replace beliefs with conscious choices and eventually reside in being versus doing. Any action they take is inspired, intuitive, and joyful. They live by the direction of something much greater. This doesn't look a certain way. Any belief that it does is a limitation.

So let go of the judgment and let go of the belief of what anything should look like and appreciate how it is. Because it is, dear one. Open your eyes. See that all beliefs are constructs and all constructs are limitations.

Oh, and by the way, all constructs are creations. But we will leave that for a different chapter.

The Belief "I Can Do it on My Own"

Many clients who I work with have the belief that they don't need help. Especially if they are in the coaching industry themselves. There's a resistance to working with someone because they don't want to be told that they're wrong and there is a desire not to look bad or be vulnerable.

I used to feel this way and thought I had to know everything. I had this belief that I had to be right and know it all. It was a heavy burden that limited my growth. Only when I was able to connect with a mentor who was willing to tell it to me straight did my growth shoot through the roof.

When I first met Lauri she just laid it all on the table. Where I was stuck, what bullshit beliefs I had about myself, and where I was still working through mommy issues. My ego reacted immediately and said, "Screw her. I don't need her telling me about my business." But then I realized that she was right. About everything. I did have hitches, I did have issues, and damn it, those were things I wanted gone. So I put on my big girl pants and went back for some more.

It wasn't easy facing the emotional hairballs that wanted to stay buried. But over time, I got used to it. She showed me that she would go to the wall with me and never let me be small. And she never did. I opened up to being wrong, a lot. The more I got used to being told, hey, this is where you are seeing the world from this perspective and it's bullshit. (Lauri cusses like a sailor) the more I was able to move beyond them.

So take a moment and ask yourself the question, Am I open

to receiving positive feedback in my life? Am I willing to hear someone tell me what I could do better and point out where I'm wonky? Am I willing to let go of my perspective and consider another? Am I attached to being right? Am I resistant to having a mentor or guide because I feel I have to know everything? If the answer is yes, it is worth resolving this and getting a mentor who can help you see things from a different or higher perspective. One who will tell you when you're full of shit or something needs to be let go of.

It's hard to see things from only our perspective, we have blind spots. When I chat with people who are interested in moving beyond their imitations the first thing I ask is, "Do you have a mentor?" Someone you can talk to, who will hold you accountable and stand for your growth? It is important to have someone who will be honest and hold up the mirror and reflect back to us our hitches and our beauty. It's important for everyone to have someone they can go to and be completely open, completely honest, completely vulnerable, and receive feedback in a way that is beneficial and helpful. This leads to authenticity and deeper connections with others.

A good mentor or guide can help us break down our negative thoughts, limiting belief structures, false realities, false personality structures and allow us to be authentically who we are. My greatest growth has come from having a mentor in my life who I know will not hold back and stands for my growth and wellbeing and will tell me when I'm being stupid and hold space for me every step of the way.

These relationships are never one-sided. They always evolve. There is always growth on both sides. When Lauri is working with me she is working through her own hitches. Through the law of attraction, when I work with my clients I always get insights. I learn about myself from others. A unique mutual receivership exists in a mentor situation. Often we look at the mentor as someone who is better than or knows more than us, but this is not so. A good mentor will tell you straight away that there is no better than, simply different experiences that we have to learn and grow through and different levels of awareness. When we share those experiences and learn from each other we lift each other up and we both grow. It's a two-way street.

You are you and I am me, and we come together for mutual benefit. We both learn and grow through the process. It requires mutual vulnerability and guts on both parties. It requires a lot for a coach to point out a bullshit belief and tell you you're being stupid. And it takes a lot for the person to receive that information and be able to integrate it. When you strip away the meaning it makes it easier to receive the message. Just because you're being stupid doesn't mean you are stupid. Would you rather be stupid unconsciously or would you rather someone point it out to you?

Many people stop mentoring because they feel stupid; they feel like their mentor is telling them the same thing over and over again. Lauri told me to stop judging alcohol for a year and finally one day I threw my hands up in the air and said, "You've been telling me this for a year!" before I finally let go of the judgment.

So consider it. Ponder it. And if it resonates with you, intend to find a mentor or guide who is right for you. You can also visit www.daniellebrooks.com for a variety of resources and mentors with diverse backgrounds from which to choose.

Separation: The One Belief That Gives Rise to All Other Beliefs

Lastly, let's talk about the big kahuna. The one belief that without it, all other beliefs crumble.

Let's talk about the belief in separation. When you believe in separation you believe that you are separate from God or Source or the Divine. You believe you are a separate individual and you are separate from all things and the world around you. You believe you have a skin that separates you from the outside world and keeps all your organs inside. But no matter how many scientists have tried, not one has actually been able to find this thing called matter.

> **MEDITATION:** Lay down flat on the floor in utter stillness. Breathe in through your nose for a count of four, pause for a count of four, release the breath through the nose for a count of four, and pause for a count of four. Do this twelve times paying particular attention to the pauses in between breaths. Then let go of the breath and just be. Don't disappear. Stay aware as you let go and relax every muscle in your body. Let go. Let go. Let go. Become aware of your vibrational nature. Where do you end and where does the outside world begin?

We are experiencing a shared dream of separation. As you cultivate awareness and become accustomed to that which you are beyond your thoughts, beliefs, emotions, and identity, the dream will cease. It is actually your belief in separation that makes it real. This was one of the hardest beliefs for me to let go and I had to actually experience it in a meditation before it was dislodged from my body. If you would like to let go of this belief, intend it. Ask for help from your guides or mentors. Ask for clarity and it will come.

You, dearest beloved being, are your own universe. There is no outside, no inside, and no center. Whatever appears to be outside of you and comes to you as perception is actually you. You are the initiator, the receiver, and the interpreter of all perceptions. You are the mountains, the oceans, and the wind. You are the plants, the animals, and all of the humans. You are the stars and the galaxies; you are what exists beyond time and space. Dissolve all borders in your meditations and experience things as they are. You are an extension of the one I Am. Sovereign, individual, and simultaneously one with All That Is.

In order to transcend the belief in separation you need to replace that belief with the truth about what you are. And this can only be experienced. I cannot give you any descriptors. But I can say, if you are ready to let go of everything, and you are willing to consider and accept that everything in separation is made up, you can use this understanding as a tool to go beyond the mind. Then you'll have liberating experiences that transform your daily life as a human. These are moments of enlightenment that take place beyond time when you let go of all your notions, all your beliefs, expectations, and dogma. You cultivate awareness and let go. You stand in the middle of the fire and burn it all down and see what happens.

As you let go of expectations of how your journey will unfold, as you go to awareness and experience moments of enlightenment beyond time, what happens in time will change. You will know experientially that everything in separation is false. The idea of being a separate individual is replaced by the experience of being an entity which exists undivided within pure consciousness. In other words, pure consciousness is aware of itself as you. This has to be realized on a deep level. At some point it's undeniable. Then you just surrender. What do you surrender to? Who you really are.

INTEGRATE: Please stop here. Being exposed to this information has begun the process of disidentification with yourself as a limited separate being and has given you the opportunity to look at yourself quite differently. Sit with this information. Ponder it. Put it in quarantine and ask questions, such as "Is this true?" See if you can experience it for yourself. Ask for the truth to be revealed. Intend it and it shall be so.

Return to your Truth Cards and create some new ones that reflect what you have realized about yourself. Be certain that you are complete and integrated with this information before moving on. If you don't feel complete with any of this information, return to the previous chapters and ask your mind to bring you more clarity. It loves to be told what to do.

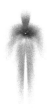

CHAPTER 7:

EMOTIONS, PART ONE

Quick Recap: In the previous chapter you learned methods in which to question beliefs and how to dissolve them. Pretty cool, huh? You learned about the Six Phases of Change and identified where you are in the process of change. You discovered how to change your beliefs so you are not in conflict with the changes you wish to make. You learned how to change perspectives. You had an insight into what life looks like beyond all constructs and are starting to get a feel for who and what you are as the aware presence that articulates your physical form. We talked about the importance of getting the help of a mentor who is willing to tell it like it is. You did a meditation designed to experience yourself as connected to all things. Most importantly you learned that the belief in separation gives rise to all other beliefs. You, dearest beloved being, are your own universe.

Now let's delve into emotions.

Emotions Get in the Way

Emotions, like beliefs, may get in the way of letting go of what no longer serves you. They can also be real buggers when it comes to living a peaceful, balanced life. Emotions LOVE drama. When you become the observer, you may witness the eruption of some powerful emotions. Your ego may want to cling to the belief that you don't have time, or other stories, such as, "It's too hard," "I can't," or "Who am I to wake up?" You may feel a strong and chaotic compulsion to eat, drink, or avoid your emotions by watching TV or scrolling endlessly through social media.

Recall from the previous chapters that 80% of most people's thoughts are negative and untrue, and 95% of those thoughts are repetitive, therefore thoughts cannot be trusted. When a thought arises over and over again it becomes a belief structure, that's what beliefs are, thoughts that you have bought into. So if thoughts can't be trusted, beliefs cannot be trusted either. In addition, emotions are what arise from our thoughts. So, if thoughts and beliefs are unreliable, so are emotions! This is crazy intense, right?

Emotions Bring Information

Emotions are what arise in response to your thoughts and beliefs about yourself and the world around you, and they are very valuable in helping you to understand exactly where you are. For instance, if you are angry, you are most likely doing something you'd rather not do. If you are bored, the boredom could be an indication that you may need more excitement in your life. Emotions bring the gift of insight in the form of triggers that tell you where you still have work to do; where you are still judging, comparing, competing, or falling into the trap of fear, frustration, insecurity, anxiety, worry or guilt and shame.

Emotions bring you information that tells you about yourself. If you feel good then you are in alignment with your true self. If you feel bad, you have some story of lack and limitation that needs to be looked at. Emotions are very valuable signposts that tell you where you are and show you what you have created via your thoughts.

Just because you have an emotion doesn't mean that's who you are. Many people say, "I am so angry." No. You are experiencing anger. The "I Am" presence within you is not limited to anger or any emotion. If you observe an emotion, it cannot be you, and all emotions are observable. You are the observer, the experiencer of the emotion, and the discerner of what the emotion has to tell you. Emotions bring you information and it is your job to decide what to do with the information they bring.

If you are driven to avoid your emotions with TV, social media, food, alcohol or drugs, you are avoiding valuable information about yourself and your life. When you look at it from this perspective you see that emotions are nothing to be afraid of. Sure, they can be uncomfortable, but what you will discover is that the thoughts that trigger your emotions are based on the past and therefore not true or necessary now. This discovery and awareness helps you process emotions from the past and let them go. Emotions bring information, but that doesn't mean the information is always reliable.

Emotions are Your Body's Reaction to the Mind

This is very important so I'm going to say it again: emotions are your body's response to the mind. For instance, having a negative thought releases certain chemicals that trigger an emotional response. Then, when you feel that emotion, it can reinforce the thought, which intensifies the emotion and reinforces the thought in this never-ending feedback loop. To get out of this awful experience, you can drop out into ice cream, TV, drugs, or social media. Sound familiar? You could also just face your emotions and learn from them. The choice is yours.

This feedback loop becomes apparent when opportunities for change and growth come our way. For example, if you have a job interview and you think, I won't get the job, the thought releases chemicals in your body that stir up the feelings of fear, rejection, and unworthiness, which reinforces other negative thoughts, which triggers even more emotions and the next thing you know you are filled with fear and anxiety over a possibility for growth and expansion in your life. The important thing to grasp is that any suffering in this instance was created by a thought or belief, which triggered an emotion that is often not based on reality.

Emotions are your body's reaction to the mind and if you don't like how you feel, ask the mind to bring you something better.

Again, I want to reinforce that you are a powerful creator and you create with your thoughts. This is but one example of how that happens. Someone once said to me that fear and faith ask the same thing; to believe in that which is unseen. Which of these two things have you experienced more of? Fear or faith?

The Difference Between Feeling an Emotion and Becoming Emotional

The difference between feeling an emotion and becoming emotional is the attachment of a story. When we don't attach a story, or buy into one, the emotion flows through us and out of us.

Here are two examples of what I have experienced in my own life:

Storytime: I was at a party once and saw a beautiful woman who looked like she had it all together. Seeing her triggered an old pattern of judgment, comparison, and unworthiness within me.

I immediately compared the two of us and found myself lacking. (Attachment of story: she's beautiful; I'm lacking) This released chemicals that brought forth the emotion of fear of unworthiness, which triggered more thoughts of unworthiness, which triggered more emotions and discomfort. I was in a loop. I responded by mentally calling her a bitch in an effort to make myself feel better. (She may be beautiful but I'm kind.) I believed the thought that triggered an emotional response and attached a story.

I have also experienced the same situation where I remained alert and aware that I was triggered by an old pattern. I increased my awareness of what was happening inside me: my mind had a thought that triggered an emotional response and I rode it out. I felt the emotion of fear of unworthiness well up inside me and move through my body and out of my body. I then shook it off and got on with my day. I didn't respond or buy into the thought; I didn't try to manage, suppress, or avoid the feeling. I did not identify as unworthy or attach a story either. I witnessed it for what it was: a thought that stemmed from past experiences that was turned into an emotion by me.

The gift of the emotion in this case was the awareness that my mind was still caught up in the pattern of comparing and judging. This gave me the opportunity to explore the pattern of unworthiness and unwind it. Now, it's important to mention that this didn't happen overnight. Each time the story arose I had to see it and let it go. Each time I did this the story unwound until it eventually faded away over time. It took awareness and letting go. Awareness and letting go. Awareness and letting go.

Whenever you experience an emotion, it is ALWAYS about you and your experience. Always. Never is it about anyone else.

Emotional situations leave an imprint on your emotional body. Some are so strong you do everything you can to not face them. Many people believe facing their emotions is like facing death. It can certainly be scary the first time you do it, but you don't die. That's just a story the ego likes to use to avoid discomfort.

If you enter into anger or any other emotion WITHOUT a story, the emotion becomes power; the power becomes your original nature, which is love, every time. For example, anger is the result of love. It is energy for defense of something you love when it is threatened. If you feel hurt, sad, or depressed, and allow yourself to feel these emotions fully, you may experience a knowing that all you really want is to love and be loved.

If you enter into anger WITH a story, it's focused on something else. Now there is blame. You did this, and that is why I feel this, this is how you made me feel, and you enter into an endless realm of action and response that goes on and on.

- Feelings are not personal. For example, peace, love, joy, and beauty are feelings. You feel them.

- Emotions are feelings with the attachment of a story. They are personal and made by false identities that you think are you. For example, fear, worry, sadness, and despair all have stories attached, do they not? I am a loving person can also be a false identity when the feeling of love is attached to a story of you as a good person.

- Becoming emotional will wrap you up in the traps of the thinking mind.

- Feeling your emotions deeply will bring you home to yourself. Your feelings become your teacher.

Can you see the difference? Many people avoid feeling. They create these huge stories and beliefs that emotions should be avoided at all costs. But when you pull back the curtain, they are like a friendly little mouse trying to keep you safe.

In one of my meditations I became aware of how I would compare myself to others and often either find myself lacking or doing all right. I felt the energy around this comparison and stayed with it for a while. I explored it like a Rubik's Cube, turning it every which way, looking for a solution. I was curious why my worthiness or lack of worthiness was dependent on comparing myself to others.

I brought to my mind's eye one person I compared myself to and I sat with that energy. I felt my way into the essence of myself and into the essence of the other person and curiously explored, and this is what I received:

"I am where I am. You are where you are. Thus the two of us meet in equal exchange."

I realized that with each exchange not only did I give something to that person, but they gave something to me. Whether it was a reflection of that which lies within myself in the form of judgment, a remembrance of something I had lost in myself like confidence, or something I enjoyed about myself. Reflections aren't always negative. And they, in turn, had an opportunity to see themselves reflected in me. Every encounter was, indeed, an equal exchange.

I then, in my mind's eye, brought in people who I have had difficulties with, or who I connect with in love—my integration clients, teachers, students, family, friends, etc.—and as I brought each one into my awareness and explored my relationship with each individual I realized the truth of this statement. "I am where I am. You are where you are. Thus the two of us meet in equal exchange." My most challenging relationship became my greatest teacher, giving me insights about myself. Whether we acknowledge it or not, each and every interaction, every day, is a gift of equal exchange. Thus, the questions beg to be asked, "What are you giving?" and "What are you receiving?"

Whatever you experience in relationship with another, it is ALWAYS about you and your experience. Always. Never is it about anyone else.

Your emotions give you the opportunity to explore this equal exchange and learn about yourself and the stories you have created, as well as the things you may be allowing or doing that you'd rather not do. Every negative thought your mind thrashes you with, every limiting belief you buy into is just a story. Every single one. Including the stories you have created about others.

What is one story you have created about your worth and value? Write it down.

When did this story first arise?

How did it serve you? Did it keep you safe? Propel you onward? Give you strength?

Do you still need that story today?

What would your life look like, who would you be without this story? What would you experience?

Here's another example of how emotions can teach us about ourselves: When it comes to food, the urge to eat may arise when your physical body is not hungry. The emotion of wanting to feed, soothe, or avoid an emotion may be strong. You may feel chaos and compulsion and experience feelings of being out of control.

- If you let the emotion well up and simply experience the emotion with curiosity, it will flow through you and out of you. *You feel the emotion.* You can even be curious and ask questions such as, "What am I avoiding? Soothing? What am I really hungry for? What could I reach for instead?" This helps you to get at the root cause of emotional eating and start unwinding it.

However,

- If your mind gets caught up in the emotion and creates a story that you deserve it, or that you'll start eating better tomorrow, or screw it, you don't want to live that life anyway, then you've gone unconscious and become emotional. *You avoid the emotion* and are driven into that bowl of ice cream to avoid the discomfort. But the discomfort is only relieved for a moment until the ice cream is gone and you start beating yourself up...again. There are many stories created here:

  - "I deserve it."

  - "I'll start tomorrow."

  - "I don't want to live that life anyway."

  - And afterward, the stories of "I can't" or "It's hard" are born.

Here's the crazy thing about the discomfort most people must face when dealing with their emotions: they are already uncomfortable. It's just that the discomfort they know is less scary than the discomfort they don't know.

Do you see the difference between feeling an emotion and getting emotional?

We can use our stories to keep us down or lift us up. *If there was no story there would be no creation!* The question is do you like what you are creating?

MEDITATION: Sit quietly for 5 minutes and wait for an emotion to arise. It may be discomfort or frustration. Your mind might create a story that the exercise is ridiculous and tell you to get up and release chemicals that give the experience of discomfort or agitation. What arises? Is there a story that your world will fall apart if you do nothing? Just identify the emotion and feel it fully. Pay attention to any story that is attached to it and ride it out while cultivating awareness. What information is it giving you? Is this information valuable? Is it true? Is it time to ask for new information? Watch as the emotion dissipates with your aware attention.

INTEGRATE: Stop here and integrate the information that has been revealed to you about yourself and the emotions you experience. Ponder it. Question it.

Recall that there is a rhythm of integration

1. Realize a new layer of all of you.
2. You settle and integrate. You get used to it, let your mind accept it, adopt it, embody it.
3. Realize a new layer of all of you.

This process has many highs, where you get insights, downloads, or restructurings of your belief systems. It also has lows that are extremely uncomfortable as you face and feel the emotions so they can be processed out of you. Be patient and compassionate with yourself as you process your emotions. Know that after you face your first emotion and ride it out without attaching a story it gets easier because you know you won't die. The relief after it is done takes weight off your shoulders.

Integration is the tears that fall when you face the sadness that was never expressed in your youth. The anger of being stuck in a construct of your making. The anxiety of not knowing what will happen if you let go of old beliefs. Be willing to look at yourself, your habitual ways of thinking and being with openness and curiosity and be courageous enough to face what arises. What lies beyond the distortions is freedom. While I can dangle that carrot before you, you must trust the process and discover this for yourself. Can you trust that what you will experience of yourself is worth the discomfort?

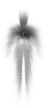

CHAPTER 8:

EMOTIONS, PART TWO

Quick Recap: In the previous chapter you learned that emotions bring you information that tells you about yourself. If you feel good then you are in alignment with your true self. If you feel bad, you have some story of lack and limitation that needs to be looked at. Emotions are your body's reaction to the mind and if you don't like how you feel, ask the mind to bring you something better. You learned the difference between feeling deeply and getting emotional and what it's like to experience a feeling without a story attached. If there was no story there would be no creation. The question is do you like what you are creating? You can tell by the way you feel. If any of this chapter feels incomplete, return to it and ask for clarification. You may find it between the words if you allow your mind to bring it. The mind does love being told what to do. Did I mention that? There is also a peaceful pause while you wait for the information to come to you that is delicious.

Emotions Are Not Your Enemy

As you begin to peel away the layers of what you are not, your mind may decide it doesn't like the change and try to sabotage you. This can happen when you do something that makes your mind uncomfortable. The mind creates a thought, taps into an old belief, and triggers an emotion. If you are not alert, it could stir up chaos and confusion as a tactic to get you to return to old behaviors and patterns. The mind is very clever. But this doesn't mean your mind or your emotions are your enemies. While it may be tempting to demonize the mind and emotions, they actually have your best interest at heart. They just want you to avoid pain and seek pleasure.

Emotions help you to realize how clear and honest you are with yourself. When you are dishonest and believe the negative stories and beliefs of the thinking mind, you feel badly. When you let those go and tap into your being, your true essence beyond all that, you feel good.

Here is a quote from the book *Althar - The Crystal Dragon* by Joachim Wolffram that I have memorized and found so helpful in giving me courage to face my emotions: "Be so bold as to face any emotional situation that shows up in your life. They know they are not real so they come forth to argue, negotiate, and fight. When they show up, expose them to pure consciousness.

This is true compassion. You don't judge, you just see them as they are; they stem from old experiences that were transformed into emotions by you." They are creations.

I highly recommend all of Wolffram's books. I find them to be valuable and experiential guidebooks for embodied ascension.

Emotions Are Nothing to be Afraid of

Facing your emotions can be scary. The first time you do this it is SO SCARY because you've never been taught to sit with your emotions. And it can feel equivalent to looking into the face of death.

It's normal to feel fear when you first begin to explore your emotions. You may feel that, like Pandora's box, once you open the door you won't be able to shut it. We falsely believe that if we fully feel our emotions, they will engulf us and we might die. So we suppress them, avoid them, and store them away inside of us. This can be what makes us sick. Many people believe that suppressing emotions is what causes dis-ease in the body.

Emotional Hairballs: As a child if you were told repeatedly that you had to work hard to succeed, the thought pattern and belief structure "I must work hard to succeed and get love or be enough" becomes an energy form that is lodged within you. When that one thought takes possession of the mind, it can take control and become your whole universe.

As you cultivate awareness, simply be aware that certain emotions may arise to be released from the physical body and it's okay. If the urge to cry arises, cry. You may find yourself crying and you have absolutely no idea why. You may find yourself in the car screaming at the top of your lungs. This is a very good sign the embedded pattern is unraveling and being released from your body. You are hacking up an emotional hairball.

I had this experience around my throat chakra. Growing up in a household of five kids I felt I didn't have a voice. When I did voice my opinion it was shut down rather quickly by my mom. This created the belief that what I had to say didn't matter and that it wasn't okay to speak my truth. Then one day I was with my partner and I was experiencing an overwhelming feeling of love and I just couldn't get it out. I was afraid. He noticed what was happening and intuitively placed his hand to the back of my neck. This helped the energy move out of my throat. The sound that I made sounded literally like a cat hacking up a hairball. While not that romantic, and quite embarrassing, it helped me hack up the fear of speaking truth.

Releasing emotional hairballs is sometimes not pretty. It often involves tears of sadness or sorrow. It involves facing the need to control, worry, or anxiety in order to process them out of you. But the feeling of relief afterwards is immense. Letting emotions, such as anger, fear, and despair, flow through you and out of you may seem very scary at first, but when you succeed at it once, you gain confidence. You discover you won't die and it actually feels quite good to let your emotions come and go without a story attached to them. Many compare it to the feeling of poison leaving the body.

So know that while facing emotions can be very scary, it is

not something you can't handle. I promise you that you won't die. In fact, after you've done it a couple times and watched an emotion move through you and out of you, it actually can feel quite good and leaves you feeling lighter and less burdened as a result.

Emotions are Only as Big as You Allow Them to Be

The truth is that when we are conscious of our emotions, when we don't obsess or dramatize them, even the most painful and difficult emotions can subside relatively quickly.

Just like thoughts, emotions are actually very small when compared to the vastness of who you are beyond your thinking mind. An emotion, when felt with attention and curiosity instead of taking you over and driving your behavior becomes something that comes and goes quickly with minimal discomfort.

I don't intend to minimize how big your emotions may feel to you, as they can feel powerful, but this power only manifests if given space, energy, and attention to do so.

Sometimes it may feel like you are possessed by a strange emotional entity that just wants to end the suffering with a bowl of ice cream, a glass of wine, or binge watching a show. Emotions have a certain energy, especially when they are attached to a story. But this doesn't mean that they can't be handled.

REFLECTIVE MOMENT: What are the top three emotions you experience daily?

1.

2.

3.

What do these emotions say about the quality of your life? Are you happy with these emotions?

What three emotions would you like to feel on a daily basis?

1.

2.

3.

Okay, good. Now, transitioning from the emotions you don't want to the ones you do want typically happens in two steps.

The first step is letting go of the emotions you are entrained to feel every day.

The second step is consciously choosing how you want to feel and adapting or integrating that feeling into your everyday life.

Consider yourself a computer who has simply been programmed to feel a certain way based on what your parents taught you, past experiences and interpretations of those events. Once you let go of an old program you have the opportunity to insert a new program.

Remember, you are an infinite creator and choosing the feelings you want to experience every day is part of the "I AM a particle of God" package. But the how to be an infinite creator instruction pamphlet has been hidden from us until now.

So step 1 is to rocket launch the old pattern from your biology. Let's talk about how to do just that.

Allow Your Emotions to Flow Through You

The best way to handle even the most monstrous of emotional flare-ups is to allow them to happen. Once they are felt fully, they will leave. Then, you can begin to decipher the message they brought you. When you feel anger, see if it is possible to really feel the anger, and even to express it fully for a couple of minutes.

You might say, "Arg! I feel so angry!" If someone asks, "Why? What's wrong?" Just say, "I don't know, I just feel this way. And it feels good!" This is liberating.

Here is an amazing strategy for handling emotions.

Emotional Mastery: The 5-Step Dissipater

Step 1: Identify the Emotion: What is the emotion you are feeling? Anger? Fear? Boredom? Frustration? Hatred? Jealousy? Sadness?

Step 2: Locate it: Once you identify the emotion, locate it. Where does it live in your body? Is it in your chest? Your throat? Your belly? Is it all over? Does your heart beat faster, does your throat close? Does your stomach turn?

Step 3: Feel It: Once you identify the emotion and locate it, feel it fully. Let it wash through you. Anger, fear, and pain are all a part of the human experience and when we suppress them they can get hung up in the body and create emotional imprints. It's when we face them, feel them, and let them go that they can be released. Emotions truly just want to be felt and then let go. If the emotion is located in the throat chakra something may need to be said or expressed aloud to release it. Ask, "What needs to be said that has not been said?"

Step 4: Let it Go: If the previous steps were done in awareness, when you get to this step the emotion is often already gone. If it's not already gone, increase your awareness and observe the emotion with curiosity. You may have attached a story to it and be caught up in the drama or pain around the emotion. Release the story, increase your awareness, and take some slow deep breaths releasing on the exhale and watch the emotion dissipate. It is very important to know the emotion always dissipates. This is not a long, drawn-out experience of dwelling in old painful emotions. It can be done in as quickly as 30 seconds. You can even observe it come and go by saying aloud,

"Emotion arising.... emotion dissipating."

Step 5: Receive the Gift: After the emotion has flowed through you, ask questions:

1. When did this first arise?
2. How did it serve me? Did it keep me safe somehow? Make me stronger?
3. Do I still need this today?
4. What is the gift of this emotion? What is it trying to tell me? What am I learning about myself in this now-moment?

Wait for the answers to come as experiential knowings. You may learn how your emotions have kept you safe or made you stronger, or formed your character, or are telling you that you are doing something you'd rather not do. There is always a gift to be received. Always.

This is alchemy at its best. When you feel your emotions, understand them, and rise above them in gratitude for how they served you, it transforms them from something to be avoided at all costs, to something of great value. You know you have used this technique properly when you experience relief, gratitude, and even joy for what your emotions have taught you.

Very important! Don't go back and look for that emotion to see if it's gone. Many people will release an emotional hairball then go back and pick it up again. Don't do this. Let it go and trust that it is gone.

Be compassionate with yourself as you face your emotional hairballs and let them go. When you get hooked or go down the rabbit hole, just say to yourself, "Oops! I went down the rabbit hole!" as soon as you realize you disappeared. Place your hand on your heart and say, "Thank you for the well intentions of these emotions to keep me safe or help me grow."

There are situations in life when we experience pain. Life happens. We all experience stress, rejection, boredom, frustration, anger, disappointment, and failure. We all experience sickness, injury, and aging. We all face death. The basic human emotions we repeatedly experience throughout our lives are inherently painful. It does us no good to avoid them, push them away, or pretend they do not exist. They are a part of us and make us who we are. When we are open to witnessing and experiencing all of our beautiful emotions, this is when we fully experience life.

The more you practice sitting with your emotions and exploring what they are trying to tell you, the more you will discover about yourself. The more small victories you will have and the more you will learn emotions are nothing to fear. In fact you look forward to them as gifts that teach you who you are and where you are in relation to yourself.

Another way to handle emotions when they arise is to simply increase your awareness that you are having an emotional experience.

Storytime: Between 2018 and late 2019 I sold my business, left a relationship, and moved to a new state. I settled into my new home and was unpacking, arranging, and putting things away. I worked in silence and found myself feeling a variety of emotions. One moment I felt excited and ready for what was ahead of me, and on the other hand, I felt lonely and afraid.

I experienced fear, and all the old thoughts that used to haunt me came rushing back in. "You don't know enough. What are you doing? I can't believe you left everything behind. You can't do this." I experienced overwhelm. I experienced frustration. I experienced a sense of disorientation and intense fear and self-doubt.

Each time an emotion arose, I used the 5-Step Dissipater, and each time one emotion dissipated another arose in its place. I was being bombarded by my ego with all the old negative thoughts, limiting beliefs, and stories that kept me stuck in the past. I felt myself shrinking and tears filled my eyes. I was getting sucked into old patterns that I thought I had already conquered. I felt the hero of my journey fall to her knees.

Feeling disoriented and in a state of severe self-doubt I reached out to my mentor Lauri who guided me out of it. She told me my ego was being a bitch and trying to pull me back into old ingrained patterns and belief systems. She had me label the emotion aloud as it arose. I said, "Self-doubt arising. Uncertainty arising. Frustration arising. Fear arising. Loneliness arising." And when I got caught in the emotion and started to cry, she snapped me out of it by saying, "Nope, you got hooked, you believed it. Do it again."

It took about 30 minutes for her to get me off the ledge.

This gave birth to a new strategy.

Emotions Arising

This strategy can be used alongside or in addition to the 5-Step Dissipater or when you've gotten snagged by old patterns and belief systems.

1. Identify the emotion.
2. Feel it rising within you.
3. Label the emotion as it rises with detachment. For instance, "Fear arising."
4. Watch the emotion go and say, "Fear leaving."

When you get emotional, you know you've been snagged. When you can label the emotion aloud with detachment, feel it rise and fall within you, you have successfully navigated an emotional hairball.

To clarify: we are not suppressing, resisting, or avoiding the emotion; we are watching it arise and leave. It's very similar to The 5-Step Dissipater energetically.

The important thing to experience is the energetic difference between getting snagged by the emotion and witnessing it.

- Getting snagged by the emotion feels like the energy of the emotion has grabbed you and taken you on a journey of a story. The energy of the emotion gets hung up within you and it feels like you are a dog chewing on an emotional bone. The important thing to note is that you disappeared into the emotion.

- Detaching from the emotion enables you to or witness

the emotion without getting caught up in its energy or story. You watch the feeling move through you and out of you. Not good, not bad, not true, or not right, or not wrong, it doesn't mean anything about who you are.

Cultivating Awareness is Key: I think I have said this before. ;-) The most important detail in both of these strategies is to cultivate awareness. The more aware you are of your experience, the more you step into your seat as the observer of your experience. This takes the wind out of the emotional sails.

Lauri taught me that what I was doing was facing my dark side. Facing my shadow. She laughed when I said, "Well, isn't that supposed to be a big deal? This seems too easy."

She said, "No. It's not true that facing the darkness within us needs to be a mighty battle against good and bad, with drama and difficulty. No. Facing your darkness, your shadow side, or the emotions you avoid truly can be as easy as saying, 'Fear arising,' 'Fear leaving,' and moving on with your day."

After we hung up, I laughed, took a deep breath, and went about my day. And every time my ego served me up an old lie, I transformed it to truth by saying, "Self-doubt arising" and then as I watched it go, I said, "Self-doubt leaving." Each time I got more confident. Each time I developed self-trust. Then one day that self-trust transformed into self-love.

Self-love is the result of facing your emotions.

You will receive many ways to work out the embedded emotions within your physicality throughout this book because not one way works for all people. Take the method that works for you and use it. The most important thing is to actively face the distorted emotional hairball so it can be released and you can find peace.

Acknowledge the emotion. Let it come on. Feel it. Look at it. Watch it go. Know where it came from. Link it to a pattern, and let it go. Understanding how your emotional hairballs arose to protect you is part of the unraveling process that ends with gratitude and relief.

One day I had a craving for ice cream. I checked in with my body and I wasn't hungry. So I sat with the discomfort of NOT having it to find out what was going on. The energy of a spoiled child reared up within me and threw a tantrum. The energy felt chaotic and compulsive and got really big, and for a moment I thought I was going to die. But I sat with the discomfort anyway, and you know what happened? It slowly dissipated. Then after the discomfort was gone I was able to ask questions. Why did I want ice cream? What was that all about?

What I discovered was that it wasn't the ice cream that I wanted. I wanted to avoid the boredom that had crept into my life. I was alone and wanted to soothe myself. I wanted pleasure. I wanted to laugh more, play more, and most importantly I wanted to love more and be loved, and ice cream was one way I had learned to love myself.

I asked what I could do instead of eating ice cream and what arose was to meditate on self-love. So I sat down and brought in love; I cultivated love, opened my heart and magnified it. I worked myself into such a tizzy fit of love that when I got up, I felt so whole and complete I wanted for nothing. I went outside for a walk and waited for my stomach to growl and let me know it was hungry.

The need to soothe myself, to ease boredom, and seek pleasure and love was a huge insight that enabled me to choose more fulfilling alternatives to meet these needs. I would not have been able to choose those alternatives unless I was aware of the emotions I was feeling.

What emotions have you been feeding, soothing, or avoiding?

What are these emotions trying to tell you?

What fulfilling alternatives could you reach for that would enhance your life?

INTEGRATION: Stop here and over the next few days be very aware of the emotions that arise within you and the stories attached to them. These stories are often tied to false identities, past experiences, or the ego's need to keep you safe. Remember the difference between being emotional and feeling deeply is the attachment of a story. Get really skilled at removing story from all emotions and watching them move through you and out of you by using the 5-Step Dissipater and Emotions Arising strategies. Don't move on until you have allowed at least one emotion to move through you and out of you and you have received the gift of what that emotion has to tell you. (You can do this now by putting the book down and sitting in silence for 10 minutes. What emotion arises and dissipates? What is that emotion telling you about you?)

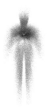

CHAPTER 9:

EMOTIONS, PART THREE

Quick Recap: The previous chapter explained that emotions are not your enemy. They tell you where you are with yourself. They are nothing to be afraid of. Even the most monstrous of emotional flare ups when faced with awareness and without story quickly leaves and dissipates. This is what I call releasing emotional hairballs; an emotion, when felt with attention and curiosity instead of taking you over and driving your behavior becomes something that comes and goes with minimal discomfort. You learned the 5-Step Dissipater, a method that teaches emotional mastery and a strategy called Emotions Arising to support you in releasing the emotional hairballs within your system. You experienced at least one emotion move through you and out of you. What did you learn from that?

If you feel complete with this information and confident in your ability to boldly face any emotion, then by all means, continue on.

Choosing and Aligning to Positive Feelings

In the previous chapter we talked about how step one is to rocket launch old patterns from your biology. This is the clearing, the purging, or the letting go of what you are not phase. Step two is to entrain yourself or adapt to the truth of who and what you really are. You're a particle of God, remember? This is not a linear process. You may go back and forth between "I am an unlimited being, nothing, and everything" and "I am a limited, flawed, unworthy human." Which of these you choose to align to more frequently and consistently becomes your manifestation. You are free to create whatever you desire and you do it by choice, self- awareness, and vibrational alignment.

Let's talk about how to do just that. In the previous section you picked three feelings you would like to experience every day. I chose joy, love, and fulfillment. But for some reason I didn't feel love, joy, or fulfillment. It wasn't until I got another bitch slap from Lauri who said, "You say you want these things but don't allow yourself to feel them. Don't ask for something if you're not willing to receive them." And at first I wasn't sure what she meant because I wanted these things terribly. Then I realized what she meant. I wasn't actively aligning to feelings of love, joy, and fulfillment on a daily basis. I wasn't feeling them. This is when I discovered that I was entrained to feeling badly. Every time I would cultivate awareness with the intent of feeling good, my ego would utterly reject the idea. Feel good? For no good reason? Why would we do such a thing? The resistance was HUGE. So instead of starting with joy, I started with gratitude and expressed my gratitude for the mundane things, like the roof over my head, the water that comes out of the faucet, and the clothes on my back. Then I reached for love. "I love sunshine, swimming, flowers, and a smile from a stranger." This enabled me to slowly work myself into feeling good. Once I was there, I was able to magnify it and actually feel the joy, love, and fulfillment and bring them vibrationally into my body and my now-reality.

Sometimes I couldn't even reach for gratitude. On those days I had to come to neutrality, or what I call the point before creation. I would empty myself of all story and identity and just be in nothing. This can be difficult for many people, especially the ones who are caught up in the routine of go, go, go and do, do, do. The idea of being still and doing nothing is uncomfortable, even terrifying. So start off small and be still for only one minute. Then as your comfort level increases, and you realize you won't die and it's actually quite relaxing, expand on the amount of time you spend in stillness doing nothing. The more you explore neutrality, the silence, stillness, and emptiness with curiosity, the easier and more comfortable it gets and you realize it's okay. It's actually quite peaceful sitting in stillness doing nothing, being empty.

MEDITATION: Set aside five minutes to sit in utter stillness. Do nothing. Be curious about this thing called the point before creation, the point before thought, idea or feeling. Can you experience for yourself that anything that comes forth from the stillness, from nothing, is a creation?

When you are empty it is easier to choose the feeling you want to experience. From a place of neutrality I would say different words and feel their vibrational impact on my body. This made it clear to me that words carry vibrational codes that trigger feelings in the body and therefore create my now experience/ reality. I chose words like peace, contentment, trust, truth, grace, and wisdom. The words you choose to play with are up to you. I encourage you to get used to feeling the words you speak and experience for yourself how they create your reality.

In the beginning I would cultivate love and allow myself to go into a state of wonderful, blissful love, then as soon as the meditation was over I went right back to self doubt. I would forget to carry the feeling with me throughout my day and it was more of a one-off meditation. But the more I stayed with it and held the intention of feeling good for the whole day, the easier it got and before I knew it, joy, love, and fulfillment were a part of my daily life. But it took work. Not work in the way we think of, but work in that I was constantly cultivating awareness of where I was, and if I was aligned to apathy and resignation I would let go, get empty, and choose consciously what I wanted to experience. It's not work; it's awareness and letting go, and choosing to align with something better.

Storytime: One day I made the decision that I would keep my heart open all day. I went into an open heart meditation and cultivated the feeling of love within me, then committed to keeping an open heart all day. I went to the grocery store and it was summertime when all of the fruits were ripe. I was literally walking through the produce department ogling and making love to all the fruits and vegetables! I would smell them, appreciate them and had a wonderful time. The produce manager saw me, came over to me, and asked if I had seen the black watermelons. I was intrigued! Really? I said, "Are they really black?"

He said, "Follow me." He took me outside to a big bin of very dark green watermelons. He explained they weren't black but a deep rich red and they were delicious. "Do you want one?" he asked me.

I said, "Absolutely" with an open heart and the excitement of a child with a new toy.

He picked one out for me and asked, "Have you tasted the peaches yet?"

"No." I said and lickety split he said, "Follow me!" We went into the store where he picked up a peach, cut it open, and gave me a slice. It was delicious! A perfect ripe peach. My heart was open and I was really enjoying the interaction. Then he said, "Oh… and the Rainier cherries!"

And all of a sudden I felt my heart clamp shut and the voice in my head said, "Quick! Get out! Run! He is going to ask you out and you will have to reject him!" I immediately said, "No, thank you. I really have to go" and beelined it out of there.

Once I was away from the produce department I stopped and chastised myself. I said, "Dani, get your ass back there and open your heart." So I did. I went back and said to him, "I just want to thank you for the work you do and the joy you bring people."

He immediately launched into a story of how he had nine lives and went into each one of them. For 20 minutes I stood there listening to him tell me the story of his life and the whole time my heart would close out of fear, and I would actively open it again. It would clamp closed, and I would open it. It would clamp closed and I would open it.

Finally, he finished his story and said, "Well, I better get back to work. It was really nice talking to you." And walked away. It was a wonderful lesson how the stories created by the mind are rarely true.

Yes, we are trained to keep our hearts closed. Entrained to fear, entrained to feeling predominantly what we call negative emotions.

I see this now all the time with my clients. They, too, have been so entrained to feeling badly that they have a serious resistance to feeling good. They don't know how to do it. This is especially true for those who are entrained to depression or anxiety. Notice how I said entrained to, not depressed people. People are not depressed; people experience depression. People are not anxious; they experience anxiety. There is a big difference. One is labeled as a false identity and another is an entrained or patterned way of being.

Recall that an emotion is the body's reaction to the mind based on past experiences. Not what is happening now. So while something terrible may have happened that caused anxiety or depression in the past, it is not happening now. To unwind this pattern we must see the situation for what it is: an emotional patterned way of being resulting from a past event that is no longer happening.

Then once the pattern has seen the light of your awareness, (it is awareness that unwinds the pattern), you can choose how you really want to feel. This is the difference between consciously choosing your state of being and unconsciously reacting to events.

Do you see the difference?

- On one hand, I unconsciously react to an event that happened in the past and carry it daily into my now-moments. I keep the story or interpretation of that event alive. I may create a victim or perpetrator story or false identity. I may create a pattern of anxiety for fear it may happen again and anxiously seek to control everyone and every experience, or I may choose to throw my arms in the air or put my head under the covers and create the story of helplessness and give up all my power.

Or

- On the other hand, I could accept that what happened happened and put it in the past where it belongs and strip all meaning from it. It does not define me. It doesn't mean anything about who I am or limit me or change who I am at my core at all. I am free now from all conditions, meanings, expectations, or attachments to the event and consciously choose the life I want to create and the feelings that daily run through me.

To repattern the mind and behaviors you must put the past in the past where it belongs and stop projecting what may happen in the future and reside in each now-moment. Each now-moment you have a clean slate. Each now-moment you can choose to feel good. You are an unlimited creator, a sovereign being. It has been said that we are so free and so loved unconditionally by our creator that we are even free to put on our own shackles and step into cages of our own making. Have you done this?

LAURI-ISM: You are so free you can choose suffering or delight and align to those choices. Many people choose misery.

Have you chosen to keep the suffering of your past alive today?

Do you have an aversion to feeling good? Are you entrained to fear, anxiety, self doubt, comparison, depression, guilt, or shame?

Knowing you've been entrained unconsciously is the first step in unwinding it and integrating the truth of who you are beyond any "programming."

Anthony de Mello, known for his spiritual writings and teachings, says, "The first thing you have to be aware of in the process of awakening is that you don't want to wake up." This speaks to the resistance to letting go of false identities of unworthiness and releasing patterned ways of being and behaving. While fear, anxiety, and depression may not serve you, they are often more comfortable than the idea that you are more than you ever imagined yourself to be.

I know, it sounds insane to have an aversion to feeling good and exploring yourself outside of limitation, but this is the way it is for many people.

The following exercise is adapted from a meditation I discovered in the book I mentioned earlier by Joachim Wolffram. This meditation is an alignment exercise that has been invaluable in helping me entrain, adapt to, and integrate higher levels of consciousness and states of being and the feelings associated with them. I have adapted it in many ways and added gratitude to the exercise because I was unable to leap to joy without gratitude as a springboard. If gratitude is too far of a reach for you, try emptying yourself of all emotion and rest in neutrality first.

Keep in mind that thoughts are vibrational frequencies that are encoded with information. When a thought has been spoken aloud its frequency and the information it contains is magnified. For instance, think of the word joy and feel into your body. Now say the word joy aloud and feel how your body responds. Its vibrational frequency is magnified, isn't it? Now think the word hate, and then speak the word hate. Can you feel how powerful it is? The spoken word is extraordinarily powerful. The information contained within the spoken word has the power to downgrade you in frequency or elevate you. It can vibrationally unlock information stored in DNA, enable you to receive downloads, upgrades, restructurings, and activate rememberings, which is what makes the following meditation so powerful.

MEDITATION: Emotional Restructuring

This is a meditation for emotional restructuring and frequency adaptation. Many people have been entrained to fear, anxiety, depression, scarcity, doubt, guilt, judgment, etc. and resist feeling good. This exercise helps you overcome that resistance and adapt to the higher frequency states of being. It can also help unwind the ego identity and integrate your true self as you get more and more familiar with the high frequency attributes of true self. Allow yourself to experience and ride the wave of high frequency emotions and levels of consciousness. This meditation holds the power to take you into a journey state without plant medicine and experience your multidimensionality.

1. Settle and Cultivate Awareness of Your True Self: Sit quietly with your feet flat on the floor, your spine straight, and your palms face up resting comfortably on your thighs. Shift your attention from your headspace to your body. Feel your feet and your entire body. Become aware of your energy, your vibrational frequency. Watch any chaos settle. Increase awareness of the aware presence that is you within the body. When you are aware of your aware presence, imagine an old fashioned round thermostat dial on the wall used to turn up the heat. This represents the level of awareness you hold. Turn that dial of awareness clockwise all the way up so that you are super aware of the sounds in the room, the fan, the creaking walls, etc. and most importantly, the aware presence that is you. Keep your eyes slightly open and downcast at a 45-degree angle to prevent you from going inward and disappearing into the meditation. You want to stay alert, aware, and fully present.

2. Become Aware of Safety: How safe are you right now? Be curious about safety. What does safety feel like? Say out loud "Safety." No one is going to hit you over the head or run you over with a car. In this moment, you are safe. When you feel safety in your body, imagine that old thermostat dial and turn it all the way up to magnify what it feels like to be safe x 1000. Let your body vibrate with the feeling of safety magnified x 1000.

3. Become Aware of Gratitude: Once you have explored and magnified safety, become aware of gratitude. If your ego is active and saying, "This is a bunch of shit," just ignore it. Say aloud, "Thank you." Focus on the small things you have to be grateful for. Think of the simple things like sunshine, the roof over your head, and a good meal. Be curious about gratitude. What does gratitude feel like in your body? When you have the feeling of gratitude, magnify it x 1000 so you are really vibrating in alignment with gratitude. Gratitude can be the gateway to these higher frequency feelings and true self-realization.

4. Become Aware of Freedom: When you are called to it, next become aware of freedom. What does freedom feel like? What does it feel like to be able to go where you want to go, experience what you want to, and express all that you are? If you need to stir up the feeling, think of a time in your life where you felt free. Say aloud, "Freedom." When you have the feeling of freedom, turn up the dial and magnify freedom x 1000! Allow yourself to spread your wings and fly!

5. Become Aware of Joy: When it feels natural, next become aware of joy. What is joy? Say aloud, "Joy." What does joy really feel like? When you have the feeling of joy, turn up the dial and magnify the feeling of joy x 1000! Let a smile cross your lips and really allow yourself to feel joy magnified times a thousand!

Stay here as long as you like.

6. Become Aware of Love: When it seems natural, become aware of love. What is love? Be curious. What does love feel like? Say aloud, "Love." When you have the feeling of love in your body, turn up the dial on love and magnify the feeling of love x 1000! What does it feel like to experience unconditional love without any reason, with no meaning, no expectations, or attachments to outcomes? Allow yourself to experience love without restraint; open your heart and let it in!

7. Become Aware of Wisdom: When the time feels right, become aware of wisdom. Say aloud, "Wisdom." What is wisdom? What does wisdom really feel like? When you have the feeling of wisdom in your body, turn up the dial and magnify it. Become aware of all the things that have happened in your life and how they brought wisdom. From this life and even past lives think of all that has happened that has brought you wisdom. Magnify it x 1000.

8. Become Aware of Beauty: Next, become aware of beauty. What is beauty? Say aloud, "Beauty." What does beauty really feel like? When you have beauty, turn up the dial and magnify it.

9. Bliss: Now combine all of these together to feel bliss! Say aloud, "Bliss" and think of the point just before orgasm! Turn up that dial and experience bliss. Really allow yourself to experience bliss! Stay in this state as long as you are called to.

10. Other Feelings: If you are called to spontaneously bring in other feelings like peace or contentment, go for it!

11. Embody the Feelings. Lastly, allow your body to adapt to the vibrational frequencies. Hold onto the feeling of bliss and let it settle within you. Stay aware; don't let the feeling go. Carry it with you as you go about your day. If you lose it, simply call it back into your awareness by saying the word aloud to trigger the feelings in your body. These feelings are always available to you; you simply have to be aware of and come into alignment with them.

You can go in any order that calls to you. If you feel like jumping from safety to wisdom, do that. There is no right or wrong way. Stay in your body at all times so you experience being both grounded and elevated.

If you have an emotional release and start crying tears of sorrow, suffering, joy, or beauty, let them come. If your body starts to shake or move in different ways, just allow it to do what it does. It's how the physical body lets go of hairballs and adapts to these new frequencies. Words are powerful. Saying, "Let go," can trigger powerful emotional releases. This is a good thing.

Wolffram calls this a light body exercise for those of you familiar with the term.

Note: Not being able to surrender, needing to control people or situations, fear, worry about what people think, fear of judgment or rejection, fear of not being good enough, guilt, and shame are all lower level ego activities with the intent to keep you safe. These are things that can cause resistance to feeling good. Thank the ego for its good intention, then elevate yourself to the higher levels where there is only love. When you get more comfortable with the elevated emotions, they will displace the lower emotions and dissolve old emotional imprints and patterns. Be patient and let whatever arises come to the surface to be processed. It is normal to experience ups and downs and highs and lows that will eventually even out over time. It is normal to experience emotional releases, intense moments of realization, and levels of expanded states of awareness. The goal is not to disappear and jet out of our physical existence, but to embody these higher frequencies and bring them here. As the saying goes...As above so below!

LAURI-ISM: The zero point is a reset that takes you back to the point before the creation of any thought or emotion. You can get back here with a breath. One breath is all it takes. An inhale and an exhale and boom! You're back to zero point. From here you can choose your intention. As you choose your intention, watch for resistance and release it to come into alignment with what you desire.

I have found the zero point to be the same as the point before creation, which brings me to neutrality, emptiness, nothing. From this point I can choose my next intention, which is a powerful place from which to intend. Never underestimate what you can do with a clear intention and an elevated emotion! Emotions are power that can enable you to experience all the different dimensions of the self.

Tips for Smoother Emotional Processing

1. If you are vibrating in fear, scarcity, or depression it can be difficult to reach gratitude. In this case, take yourself back to Lauri's zero point. Empty yourself

of all stories and come to neutrality. Then reach for a better feeling thought. Start with contentment and hope and work your way up from there. Going to joy and bliss may be too big of a leap right out of the gate.

2. The way the ego fights is through emotion. Always address the emotion without a story and the ego has nothing to grab onto. The ego knows facing your emotions is the beginning of the end of its identity, so reassure it that it will not die, but transform.

3. Know when you consistently address emotional hairballs as they arise, you work them out of your system.

4. When you learn to navigate your feelings, you won't use substances, TV, or social media to avoid them.

5. The key to processing emotions is to cultivate awareness so you are the witness of the emotion.

6. Curiosity disassociates you from the emotion. As you explore it, you detach from it.

7. Be dedicated to consistently choosing to feel good. It's not a one-off. Many people give up just when manifestation starts percolating below the surface and they fall into apathy and resignation and that becomes their reality.

8. Any time you feel constricted it's a lie. Emotions are ways to know yourself in each moment. You understand yourself and where you are based on emotional responses.

9. Attune to love. Love is a frequency. It is the activity of source, and this love is truly unconditional. When you align to and acclimate to that frequency, you become it. You can vibrate love and be love

incarnate. Love is a way of being and operating in a very high frequency. Let go of what you think love is and explore the frequency of love in meditation and your daily life.

The Entire Journey

More Balance: As you process and release emotional imprints from the body the emotional highs and the lows even out. Riding the emotional roller coaster no longer becomes the experience of riding ecstatic bliss one moment and descending into deep depression the next. Fear, anxiety, anger, and resentment fade and you may experience tinges of perhaps light sadness or melancholy instead. The emotions aren't as dramatic. Drama is the best way to describe emotions and a deep sense of peace and trust describe feelings. You become an individual who feels deeply without the highs and lows. Now when you have a bad day, the feeling is just "Meh." You become more balanced.

Self-Trust Increases: As you work through the emotional gunk, you become more trusting of yourself and your abilities to handle the emotions that arise. You know that you've come out the other side when you carry with you a constant knowing that everything is going to be okay. You trust and are content. You know that whatever arises within your field of consciousness you are capable of handling it. Self-trust becomes dominant with moments of self-love sprinkled in. One day you walk by a mirror and experience self-love and it's a surprise.

How high are your highs? How low are your lows? How much peace and self-confidence are you feeling? These are indicators that let you know where you are in relation to yourself and your journey.

Your Manifestation Skills Improve: As you fine-tune your emotional tuning fork and learn to stay in resonance with what you want, manifestation happens. It's not just a one-off. People think they can do a ten-minute meditation on abundance and go into scarcity for the rest of the day and expect that they are going to manifest abundance. No. You have to vibrate in abundance the majority of the time for the abundance to become your new current reality. You have to come into alignment with it at all levels of thought, mood, temperament, and personality.

What You Want: Most people think they want money, a partner, health, or a new job. But what they really want is what those things will give them, which is freedom, love, balance, and purpose. Ask yourself, why do I want the things I want? What will they give me? Then you will be at the root of your desires. Bring those feelings into your meditations and carry them with you throughout your day!

You Become Sovereign: The more you work through your emotions the more you realize how you feel is a choice and you make that choice every moment of every day. When you study successful people you will find that they have made a choice, a solid decision; they have chosen a North Star. For example, I will never be poor again, I will overcome, I will achieve this, I will do that. The decision was made and they processed any emotion that was not in alignment with that North Star. They expanded their belief of their personality structure out of poverty into wealth, out of self-deprecation into self-trust, and they dissipated emotions over and over and over again to bring them into alignment with that North Star. They give up any victim role and become the creator of their destinies before those destinies manifested.

You Choose Your Reality: Choice is how we create. Choice, self-awareness, and vibrational alignment via our emotional feeling self. It is a feelings game. This is nothing new. Esther Hicks has been talking about this for over 20 years. Intellectually we get this, but some of us are not willing to feel good in order to bring about what we want in life. Some of us are. Which are you?

You Feel Good: Be willing to say I will tolerate this no more, willing to say I choose this above all else, and I will choose this every day, every moment, every hour, every week, every month, and I WILL dissipate anything that gets in the way. If you do this, you will see changes in your life.

You Become Grateful: Gratitude is a feeling state that naturally arises when you release old belief structures and emotional imprints and receive the gift of your emotions. Take a moment now and say, "Thank you." Can you feel your heart open and experience an inward movement of energy? Can you feel the energy of receiving that the words carry with them? Saying thank you over and over can be very beneficial in putting you into a state of receivership.

It Gets Easier: It used to be extremely difficult to face and process emotions because we didn't know how. We were so disconnected from our emotions. There were a few people who were pioneers and breaking the way, but now it is common knowledge and the collective awareness is changing. More people are breaking through their negative thoughts and limiting beliefs and handling their emotions and transcending them. They now use high frequency feelings to create their realities. This is making it easier for the rest of us. We are one body of consciousness. Think of this body like a tapestry in which every one of us is a precious fine thread. When one person makes a change that change becomes available to the rest of the tapestry. Change is happening quicker and easier and with greater joy than ever before.

You See Your Progress: At first it may not seem like it. It may seem at times like you are forever letting go and letting go and letting go, and it may not feel like you are getting anywhere, but you are. Then one day you look back and see how far you've come. The thoughts that used to beat you up, no longer do; the beliefs you used to hold are no longer in place and your emotional roller coaster has evened out.

You Become Authentic: Looking back on my life, 2020 and 2021 were years of one big emotional release after another. I spent much time curled up in bed feeling emotions and letting them go, crying and struggling with old beliefs. Sometimes I would let one go and pick it back up again, and let it go and pick it back up again. Each time I let something go I got closer and closer to that which I am. It was difficult at first, but when you know how, releasing beliefs and emotional hairballs and false identities is not as difficult as you think. When you move through one emotion you gain confidence and you know that you can move through another, and another, and another. As you peel away the layers of what you are not, you have the opportunity to experience that which you are. You become more authentically you.

You Become Intuitive: The more you let go of what you are not, the more your channel to the divine opens and you begin to receive information. You become adept at receiving imprints, concepts, images, knowings and interpreting them; you can communicate with the quantum field.

You Come Home to You: When you release the emotional hairballs within you, you come to a place where there is nothing left to release. You find yourself in a place with no identity, no beliefs, and are aware of yourself as something much different than you imagined. You may still get triggered, but you won't react. You will just watch the trigger come and go and remain in your seat as the aware presence. Without the highs and lows of the emotional roller coaster you even out and a feeling of deep peace and contentment permeates you; you get more and more familiar with this thing called oneness and you come home to you.

INTEGRATION: You have a history of emotions. Emotions are the fuel that can take you to higher levels of consciousness and experiences of your multidimensional self. They are a force to build something better or destroy something. You've been entrained and now must go through an unknowing for freedom of choice of something new. All feelings are available to you. When you align to your choice, life moves in that direction. You have to be willing to feel good.

Read through this chapter several times before moving on and continue to use the 5-Step Dissipater and Emotion Arising strategies to release the emotional patterns embedded within you. Use the Emotional Restructuring Meditation to acclimate and align to the higher frequency emotions. Get clear as to the emotions you are entrained to and know with certainty and clarity how to entrain yourself to something new before moving on.

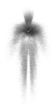

CHAPTER 10:

THE EGO, PART ONE

Quick Recap: In the last chapter you discovered that much of humanity is entrained to feeling negative low vibrational emotions. You received an emotional restructuring meditation to unwind this programing, as well as tips for smoother emotional reprocessing to align you to feeling good. You had a glimpse into the entire journey of what's available to you as you master your emotions, choose feelings consciously, and come into alignment with those choices. You got really clear as to the emotions you are entrained to and how to entrain yourself to something new.

Now let's delve into the ego.

The Ego

The ego has been studied for years. We now know the age of its inception, how it grows, and how it drives our behavior. Science and psychology have taught us how the ego arises, forms, and creates suffering and problems for humans. We also now know how to handle the ego, how it serves us, and how to transcend it.

Throughout my life I heard over and over from many different people, "The ego is a source of suffering, but you can't live without it," and each person said it with such conviction that questioning it seemed unnecessary. From psychologists to psychedelic explorers, everyone I knew held this perspective. And when I reached a certain point in my life, when I no longer wanted this ego because it was a real pain in my ass, everyone said, "Just make peace with it. It's not your enemy." Yet, when I thought of all the enlightened masters, none of them appeared to have an ego. In addition, the ego to me represented the false self, so it seemed that transcending the ego was my first order of business on my journey to enlightenment. I don't know how I knew it, but I just knew that the ego could be transcended. So I set out in isolation to quietly dissolve my ego and discover the truth of myself.

Transcending the ego became such a focal point in my life that in one of my plant medicine journeys I received the knowledge that the ego can indeed be transcended. I remember screaming at the top of my lungs, "Death to the ego!" At another point in that same journey I received the message, "The ego only serves to block the divine. You can live without it. It's why you came." When I shared this with a few people, I got skepticism. Nope, you must make peace with it was the best I got.

But I just knew the message I received was the truth so I continued on my journey to, in my own words, "rocket launch that motherfucker." I was determined to peel away all layers that I was not, all the layers of the false self that the ego represents, to get to the core of that which I am.

I quickly discovered that while peeling away the layers of what I was not sounded easy in theory, it was more difficult than I thought. My ego kicked and screamed and would have nothing to do with my idea of rocket launching it to the moon. The more I fought my ego, the worse it got. For six months I struggled and fought the ego (which I do not recommend you do) and got nowhere. The ego, I found, can be very difficult to transcend because the ego or false self will do everything it can to survive. In short, it's very feisty. The reason for this is the belief that if the ego dies, so will you.

> **REFLECTIVE MOMENT:** Think about this for a moment: if you didn't have an ego, if you didn't have any identity, no identity as mom, daughter, worker, husband, nice person, or spiritual being, who would you be? What would you experience?

If you experienced the feeling of nothing momentarily laced with a bit of fear, then you hit the nail on the head. Of all things humans face, death is right at the top of the list. So transcending the ego is one of the scariest and most difficult things a human can do. To many, it feels like dying a slow painful death as you peel away the layers of what you are not to get to the core of what you are. This is what makes it so difficult.

But you can't die. You, my dear, are immortal. You are pure consciousness. The aware presence or divine essence that resides currently in a physical body. You are infinite, timeless, unlimited, whole, complete, and utterly indescribable. Knowing this can help you make the transition of identity from ego or the limited being you think you are to the divine operating as a persona in physical form. It certainly helped me.

So instead of fighting the ego, I became super aware of my ego and constantly asked the question, "Is this true? Is this me?" I studied the ego. The birth of the ego and eventually the dissolution of false identity represented by the ego and the following is what I discovered on my journey.

The Birth of the Ego

The first thing I researched was when the ego first arrived on the scene. This has been studied extensively by psychologists and it turns out that when you were born you came into this world without an ego. You had an intuitive nature. Your level of consciousness was pure awareness and you had no identity or no sense of "I."

As a child you also had no filter and would say whatever came to mind. You would play, imagine, and create to your heart's content. You were not yet tied to an identity. You just were. You were born unconditioned and free. You were free to go where you wanted to go, do what you wanted to do, express yourself in any way you liked, and you said whatever you wanted to say. You didn't care what other people thought.

Then, between the first and second year of life, you started to recognize the different roles people played, and little by little, identification and discrimination between subject and object began. You moved from Oneness and your knowing of "Self" as awareness and connected to all things to "I am a subject, and there are objects and space between us." It is this transition from Oneness and all connectivity to a subject and an object when the ego arrives on the scene in the form of "I"

First, you experienced external objects like toys, food, and things that you liked and disliked. You took the things you liked that felt like they contributed to your sense of self and began to identify with them. This is when the world around you in the form of things, ideas, thoughts, and beliefs are no longer just things, ideas, thoughts, and beliefs, but things you have attached to, things that become a part of who you think you are. You are no longer a connected articulation of the divine, a piece of that which can never be identified or limited. You are now a separate character based on the ideas, thoughts, beliefs and rules of your parents, guardians, and the world around you. You also started to identify with material things and formed an attachment to them. Toys, clothes, and other things become identity enhancers.

Then as the ego continues to develop it reinforces its false identity with beliefs about your personality, talents, and abilities. These aspects become the structure of your personal identity. The character you call you.

For example, thoughts, ideas, beliefs, or perceptions that contribute to the ego structure or false identity are:

"Being fat is bad and thin is good."
"I am better than you because I have better toys."
"I'm not good enough unless I do these things."
"I'm not lovable unless I do these things."
"I have to look good to belong."
"I have to do this and not that to get love."
"My red hair makes me ugly."
"I can't do anything right."

> **REFLECTIVE MOMENT:** Since the ego arrives on the scene at the moment a child identifies with something, I wondered what would happen if a child maintained a sense of Oneness—a sense of connectivity with all things—and chose to experience life without identifying with or attaching meaning to anything. What would that be like?

It's an unlimited feeling just pondering it. No negative thoughts of "I can't." No limiting beliefs of, "I am not good enough." No comparisons, competition, or judgment of identity or another's identity because there is no identity, just one unlimited consciousness exploring the material realm through you and me.

For the baby born to parents who let their progeny roam without fear, the world may be a wonderland filled with amazing things.

The child who is constantly watched like a hawk for fear they will get hurt may pick up that the world is a dangerous place. If a child falls they may perceive the event as painful and startling and cry, or they may perceive it as non-painful and laugh. One event, two perceptions of the event, two personalities born. For example, when you have thoughts about yourself that you agree with, you construct a self-image within your self-awareness. This mental construct of your "self" is, of course, just a construct and is not who you are.

I was once at a store admiring a picture on the wall when the parents of the artist came by and told me the story of their son, who they decided to raise unconventionally. They decided to only teach him topics that he showed interest in. One day they were in the garage and their son said, "Quick! We need to go to Home Depot now." They recognized inspiration and hopped in the car and drove to Home Depot where he grabbed paint, brushes, and other supplies. When he got home he painted the picture that was resting on the wall. I asked if their son had learned how to read and write and they said, "Yes. He is very curious about the world." At that time he was 12 years old.

I tell this story to reinforce that we are all brought up within constructs or belief systems created by our parents and the world around us. I grew up within the construct of Catholicism which taught me I was not good enough from the get-go. If I didn't go to school, get good grades, and say my prayers, I was not a good person. Guilt and shame were very familiar to me, and for many, many years I believed that I was not good enough and never would be. Talk about a false identity! Now to be clear this was not my parents' fault; they were taught by their parents and their parents were taught by their parents. No one ever thought to question the construct.

The ego or false identity is born as a result of you taking in information about the world around you, choosing what attributes you like, rejecting the ones you don't, and attaching to those things as self. It's a persona that you create. In many ways it is a beautiful creation of your own choosing. Yes, you may have created it unconsciously, but you chose to forget in order to remember, remember?

This certainly softened my perspective about the ego. I saw that I had identified with so many things throughout my life. It wasn't the ego's fault, and it wasn't my fault either that I was caught up in a false identity of unworthiness and stories of "I can't." I mean, it's not like "Don't identify with things" is a class taught in school. I also saw that if I removed the things I had identified with, it would show me the truth of who I am, and I wanted that more than anything.

INTEGRATION: What events happened in your life that triggered thoughts, ideas, or beliefs about yourself that may not be so kind or flattering? What stories about yourself have you attached to? How was your character formed by how you perceived events and the world around you?

If you removed those things what would you experience about yourself?

The Ego is a Faculty

If you don't attach to an identity there wouldn't be an ego. There would just be a faculty called the mind bringing you information and you would be the non-attached observing presence that chooses what to do with that information. Sure, you would still have a persona called Joe, or Cindy, or Bob, but you would know who and what you are in truth.

If you're having an identity crisis right now, congratulations! Take a few deep breaths and know you're not going crazy, you are not going to die, and you are absolutely not going to live a boring life without an identity. No way. When you understand that the character you call you is not etched in stone, that it is a creation that you brought to life, and that you can mold it, change it, and craft it to be anything you desire, *and wear it loosely knowing it could never be you,* then you are free.

The ego is not an evil aspect of who you think you are. It's just a compilation of ideas, beliefs, and perceptions that you thought was you. Detach from those ideas and beliefs and you return the ego back to the faculty of the mind it originated as.

Let's say that again in a different way: The ego originated as the mind, whose job is to bring you information. When you attached to that information, and thought it was you, a false identity was born.

Again, the mind is designed to bring you information and it's your job as the aware presence to discern what to do with that information. For instance, your eyes are a faculty that bring you information about the world around you. Your nose relays information regarding smell, and your mouth is a faculty that brings you information about the food you eat. The ego is also a faculty. It is a faculty of the mind designed to bring you information in the form of thoughts and ideas, which trigger emotions. It is your job as the conscious discerner to choose what ideas and thoughts you will accept and which ones you will not, just like you decide what to put in your mouth.

When you assume your position as the aware presence, over time the false identities fall away and you retrain the mind to bring you more goodness and less crap. It returns to the faculty it originated as and becomes a faithful bringer of information. The mind quiets and becomes a useful tool that helps you navigate daily life.

The thoughts and ideas you accept are what create your beliefs, your personal reality, and your experience. For example, "Money is good" or "Money is bad." Whichever idea you discern to be true for you is what will create your beliefs, experience, and your reality.

Today, most of humanity is walking around with a limited personality structure that they think is who they are. They have completely given up their role as the discerner and let this faculty run the show on autopilot. As a result, they are literally an organic blob of habits and conditioned patterns and behaviors.

Talk about the zombie apocalypse!

If as children we were taught to discern, the ego would be regarded as a highly valued faculty, instead of an annoying false identity. The term ego would actually disappear. We would navigate the physical world in an integrated partnership with the mind. Your persona or character then becomes an articulation of the divine, an interface that allows you, as the divine incarnate, to experience physical reality.

The ego, however, doesn't like this idea of disappearing or returning back to its original role as a faculty, and in the beginning will kick and scream. It is helpful to reassure the ego it doesn't die; it transforms and you work together in an integrated partnership. The more you say no and swipe left on the information that doesn't serve you and swipe right on the information that does—just like you would swipe on the dating apps—the more the mind adapts.

I tell my clients to pretend they are Tony Stark in the movie *Iron Man* where he is at his 3D computer swiping screens left and right, totally in control of the information being brought to him. The mind loves to be told what to do. The more you say yes, no, yes, and no, and absolutely not, go get me something better, the more the mind learns, and the more space in between thoughts you will experience.

At first when you take your seat as the aware presence, thoughts and ideas about yourself and the world around you swarm like a disturbed bees nest and seem impossible to master. But for the person willing to try, eventually the bees calm down and your ability to choose your thoughts, feelings, and experience improve.

This takes cultivating awareness and asking questions such as, "Is this true? Does this information serve me?" The more you do this, the quicker any false identities you are attached to will fall away. It just takes time, awareness, and repetition as you consciously choose over and over again what is true for you. It helps tremendously to thank the mind for bringing you information and trying to keep you safe.

Storytime: Imagine that at some point in life things get tough and all you want to do is disappear. So you put this faculty called the mind on autopilot and decide to take a nap in the back seat of this thing called your physical body. You give up your seat as the discerner. Without questioning the information it brings to you, you become a passive passenger and are no longer driving the car as the creator of your reality. Your reality and your personality are now made up of thoughts, ideas, and beliefs chosen not by you, but by the faculty given control while you sleep.

The more control the faculty has the more it thinks it is you and the more it will do all it can to keep you safe. It doesn't have common sense; it just navigates in such a way to avoid pain and seek pleasure and does what it can to avoid rejection, loss or humiliation while you sleep. It looks at the world around you and compares your personality to others and either finds you lacking or doing okay. It will steer the car appropriately to keep you working hard so someday you will be good enough, or it will deem others inferior to validate that you're okay. The ego loves people-pleasing behaviors in an effort to validate itself and get love. All it cares about is getting love and approval. It doesn't care what it has to do to get it. It will tell you to close your heart, don't take a risk, and whatever you do don't speak your truth lest you will fall on your face, get rejected, look completely unlovable, and life will be over.

In other words, stay here where it's safe. Extremely boring, but safe doing what everyone else is doing. More, more, more is the mantra of the ego, which is never satisfied, never fulfilled, and forever wanting. Underneath, the intention is pure. Really the ego just wants to keep you safe, get love, and be enough. It doesn't know that you already are enough, whole and complete, and deeply loved while you nap in the back seat without a clue as to where the ego is taking you.

The thoughts "I am unlovable" and "unworthy" are information brought to you by the ego when it compared you to others, took in social constructs, and perceived things a certain way. This is information that made it into your operating systems without discernment. "I'm not smart enough. I'm not pretty enough. I'm not thin enough. I need money to be happy. I need a partner to be happy. I can't. I don't have time..." And the list goes on and on of thoughts and beliefs that made it into your operating system while you napped in the back seat.

Now after a really long nap you are waking up, stretching your arms, and wanting to take back the wheel and assume your sovereign role as the discerner, the chooser, the creator of your reality. The personality structure called you now has programmed ways of thinking and being that need to be deleted. But there is so much chaos, so many negative thoughts thrashing you, so many limiting beliefs and unruly emotions that you believe you have no control. But you do.

In addition, because the ego has had control all this time, it doesn't want to relinquish its power. It goes on red alert and kicks and screams anytime you peel away any of the negative thoughts, limiting beliefs structures, or false identities it used to keep you safe. It's scared it will die, and you are scared to die because you think the personality structure created by all the undiscerned thoughts and ideas is what you are. But that's not you. Not in a million years.

So you decide to wake up and take responsibility after your long nap. Taking back control is a matter of returning the ego back to the faculty of the mind it originated as. It is a matter of stepping back into the driver's seat as the chooser of your thoughts and beliefs and re-establishing your place as the observer, discerner, and chooser of every piece of information this faculty brings you.

Never refer to the ego again as you. The ego is NOT who you are. The mind brought you information that you bought into. You agreed to that information, identified with it, and thought it was you. The information the mind brings you about yourself is not true unless you discern it to be. The mind is a valued and treasured asset that brings you information. Your job is to DISCERN. To CHOOSE. Do you want the information it brings? Does it serve you? Swipe right. Is it unhelpful? Does the information reek of distortions of fear, self-doubt, unworthiness, and judgment? Swipe left.

The problem people have is that when it comes to demystifying the ego, removing its identity status as us, we think it's killing a piece of who we are. In many ways this is true. It's killing off a false identity. This can be very painful especially if we are attached to what we think we are. But it is not who we are. We are the amazing, unlimited, conscious presence that receives the information and chooses whether to keep it or not. We don't die. We never could. As Lauri would say. "What about being an unlimited particle of divinity do you not understand?"

The ego may present an idea of who you are or what you are not, but those are just ideas and concepts. Nothing compared to the true essence that is you.

By definition then, the ego or false identity is the totality of what you believe about yourself and pretend to be. How you perceive yourself and want to be perceived by others also plays a role.

REFLECTIVE MOMENT: What do you believe about yourself? Do you believe you are spirit residing in physical form? Or are you a flawed and limited human identity?

Whether you have created a fulfilled, joyous identity or an unworthy, unlovable identity, it is important to know that all identities are limiting and impermanent. Think about this for a moment. The false self, the ego, and even the persona you wear loosely will die when your physical form ceases to breathe. But the essence of you lives on. It is eternal. You're enjoying an amusement park trip, remember? So the question begs, "Do you like the personality structure you have created?" Are you happy with the character you call you?

We create our character most often based upon what others think or what we believe we "should" be. How do you want to be perceived by others?

REFLECTIVE MOMENT: What if others' opinions don't matter? What if there was no right/wrong, good/bad, or should/shouldn't, and you could freely do, be, have, and express whatever you like as an articulation of the divine? Better yet, let's say you have an expiration date of one year from now. What would you change?

Your Persona is an Interface

People often say to me, "Well, if I'm not worried about what others think, and I come into alignment with myself as divine, and I am completely free to do, be, have, and express whatever I like as the divine in form, what do I do?" They are paralyzed by the freedom before them. I had this experience and it is very interesting. I felt so free, I didn't like the freedom. I was so caught up in the constructs of good/bad, right/wrong that I had no idea what to do, what I liked, or what I wanted to bring forth. It took me a long while to realize that I was free to just be. Just be. To do what I wanted to without judgment. The weight of "I have to, I need to, I should, I shouldn't" lifted like a thousand pounds off my shoulders. But still the idea of should and shouldn't wouldn't leave me alone. I truly didn't know what to do without the worry of what others thought or the fear of not being good enough to drive my actions.

Then a good friend of mine, Chris Hay, posted on Facebook, "It's okay to remain unmoving until the right action arises." And that saved me. For the first time in my life I stopped. Everything. And it was uncomfortable at first, then it got easier as I relaxed into letting go of my identity as a human doing and became a human being.

I gave myself permission to do nothing, to peel away all the false identities of "Not good enough, a bad person, a spiritual person, a good person, a victim, a perpetrator, a seeker" and the list goes on and on. And with each false identity that I peeled away I came closer and closer to my true self.

My persona became an interface. The only way I can describe it in a way that you may understand is that as my conscious awareness increased, my vibration increased, I came into resonance with the divine and left my small self behind and experienced Oneness. I felt myself to be an electrical cord connected to source at one end and acting as an open door for that vibrational frequency to come into this world on the other end. I felt myself to be a permeation, connected to all things, yet individuated and without identity. Nothing. Yet everything. There was no me and there was no you...yet we shared the space between us in ways I can't describe. I know who and what I am, as something that could never be known. There are too many paradoxes to convey. It can only be experienced. If I succeed at all in describing Oneness I totally fail.

Today I know myself to be an interface, a portal for divinity to be experienced in form as me. But there is no identity. That which I am can never be identified. Yes, I have a persona called Dani and I wear this costume very loosely knowing what I am in truth. Do I fall out of alignment? All the time! Does my ego appear back on the scene from time to time? Yes. Do I have mastery under my belt? Oh...yes and heck no! Riding this thing called a physical body is crazy and there are many things it can do that I'm not even aware of. For now it's enough of a task to just be here.

Storytime: I have taken on many false identities. From massage therapist to nutritional therapist to clinical herbalist to author, speaker, intuitive eating expert, and entrepreneur to being a mentor and spiritual guide. I've played the roles of wife, lover, girlfriend, sister, aunt, friend, and identified with many things. I've been a sailor, a skier, a hiker, a world traveler, and more. I've gone from being financially successful to being dirt poor.

I've had deep rooted beliefs of not being good enough, smart enough, thin enough, and the list goes on. I've avoided difficult emotions because I did not want to face them. After all, if people saw what was beneath the roles I played they would see my fears, jealousies, anger, frustration, self-doubt, judgment, guilt, shame, and blame. They would see the monster I spent most of my life avoiding and hiding. The monster of my authentic self. So I buried the monster deep within me and pretended it didn't exist.

Then one day the monster knocked on my door and asked to be let in. It said, "Please let me in. I am part of you and I want to be seen."

At first I was afraid of what I might see and said, "No way. If I look in your eyes I will surely die."

But something gave me the courage to open the door and let the monster in. And what I discovered was that the monster was small and it cowered into a corner and was just as afraid of me as I was of it. It was covered in uncertainty. It was layered with fear, anger, guilt, shame, and all the emotions I tried so hard not to face.

I approached it slowly and one by one I cautiously began to remove each of the layers. I faced the fear and as I removed it from the monster the emotion welled up within me and I thought I would die. But I didn't. I discovered that fear is an illusion. I mean, what was it going to do? Hit me on the head?

I survived. This gave me courage, so I looked at all the emotions I felt I shouldn't have. One by one the emotions rose within me like waves and again, I felt like I would die. But I didn't.

Jealousy brought the gift of pleasure and diversity. When I stopped comparing and judging and finding myself lacking, I discovered that what I was truly seeing was something I liked, enjoyed, and admired. Anger helped me see where I wasn't being true to myself. Anger always arose when I was doing something I didn't want to do. Same with frustration. These emotions brought the gift of clarity to know when I am and am not in alignment with my true self.

Blame showed me how I wasn't taking responsibility for my life and paying the role of victim. This was a hard one to face. But again, I survived it.

As I peeled away the layers the monster got lighter. Beneath the thick coat of everything suppressed I found a scared little girl trying to stay safe, trying to get love, and I found myself looking into my own eyes. This was like looking into a mirror and at first I got angry and railed at myself for not doing the things I wanted to do, for not being strong enough, smart enough, good enough and I let the emotions fly. When the anger died down I cried. I cried at how hard I was on myself. I faced all the self-hatred that was inside of me, and again, I thought I would die. But I didn't.

After the tears stopped falling I found myself rocking back and forth comforting myself. I experienced self-compassion. Over time I got more and more courageous and looked forward to my time looking into my own eyes. The anger died down and did not return. The sadness and self-hatred also went away and was replaced with trust, and eventually one day I found myself walking by a mirror and experienced self-love.

> **REFLECTIVE MOMENT:** If you let your monster in and faced that which wants to be seen, what would you gain from the experience? Who would you be

after all the distortions are gone? Are you courageous enough to go looking?

MEDITATION: Cultivate awareness and repeat the question, "Who am I?" As thoughts and ideas arise into your awareness, let them go. Let go of everything that arises. Let go. Let go. Let go. Be with yourself. The essence of you. Experience yourself as the point before creation. The point before thought. What do you experience?

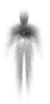

CHAPTER 11:

THE EGO, PART TWO

Quick Recap: In the last chapter you saw how the ego is born as a result of you taking in information about the world around you, choosing what attributes you like, rejecting the ones you don't, and attaching to those things as self. You learned the ego is not you but a false identity that was given the run of the show for a while. The ego when stripped of identity leaves you as the aware presence utilizing this faculty called mind. It is a paradox that we are One with all of creation, yet sovereign and individual. Therefore, you need a character on this stage of life to express, touch, taste, and feel. It is the physical character that enables you to experience and share. The secret is to wear this character loosely and not be attached to it because it will never be you. You were given several reflective moments to ponder who you are as nothing and everything. How did that go?

Let's continue on with the ego.

Dismantling the Ego

When you first understand the ego to be a faculty, it is a huge relief. Yes! The ego can be dealt with! You take back your seat as the discerner and spend the next few months diligently swiping left to reject information and swiping right if the information is helpful. Whew!

While this sounds simple, and it is, it is not easy because the ego will bring you all the same information it has brought you in the past repetitively and aggressively. What started as a valuable faculty has now morphed into an energetic entity that doesn't want to revert back to its original role.

A lot of discomfort may arise in the beginning because your ego dreads one thing most: change. So allow any resistance to come up without judgment. You are not looking to "kill" the ego, or deny its existence. You want to gradually and gently dissolve any identity and return it to the faculty it originated as. To do this, the ego must be stable. For it to be stable, you must be familiar with it, you must have compassion with it, and you must love it and appreciate it for its positive intentions. All egoic intentions are positive. Truly all the ego really wants is to keep you safe and get love. It just goes about it in rather twisted and insane ways.

The ego is your protector and has been a part of you since you were a small child to help you cope. Appreciate the ego, love it, and have compassion for it while you dis-identify from it. True compassion is the knowing that the ego is not real, and you don't make it real by focusing on it.

The Three Types of Ego

According to Joachim Wolffram there are three types of ego:

The Cancerous Ego

This is the ego (false identity) that is burdened with enough is never enough. More, more, more is the signature of the cancerous ego that will abuse power and wisdom for its own purposes. This is the ego that wants to assimilate everything in its path. More alcohol, more food, more drugs, more money, more clothes, more stuff. More, more, more, and more is never enough.

The Weak Ego

Then there is the weak ego. This is the ego easily shaken by fear, doubt, anxiety, low self-esteem, and stamina; this is the identity in danger of a mental breakdown on the path to enlightenment. Self-doubt, uncertainty, and lack of confidence are qualities of the weak ego. It needs lots of love and reassurance.

The Healthy Ego

The healthy ego can be identified as having a combination of the intuition or knowing that there is something more beyond itself. The healthy ego is the persona you operate in while in physical form that holds a false identity but not so tightly.

Sooner or later the healthy ego comes to the conclusion it cannot be what it perceives. The healthy ego perceives the body and knows if it can observe the body; it cannot be the body. The healthy ego perceives thoughts, beliefs, and emotions rising and falling within its awareness and concludes it cannot be those.

Sooner or later the healthy ego realizes that anything it perceives cannot be itself, and therefore, returns to the faculty it originated as a perceiver. A bringer of information. AKA the mind.

Unhealthy Ego Indications

The following are indications the unhealthy ego may be active and triggered:

- You experience strong emotional reactivity

- False confidence (overcompensation)

- Black and white/rigid thinking

- The need to be right

- Rejection of any idea that conflicts with the ego's beliefs

- Competition (a belief that another person's success hinders your own)

- Judgment of others or self (mocking, insulting,

gossiping, threatening); constant comparison to others

- Analysis paralysis (obsessive thoughts that stop you from completing any action)

- The need to control people and situations

- Feelings of significance above others

- Guilt or shame

- Fear designed to stop you from doing something new, speaking your mind, saying no to someone, facing an emotion, or changing a behavior

- You talk to and argue with yourself

If you look closely at your ego you will see it can be quite insane.

Other indications that you're living in reaction to the ego:

- You feel emotionally depleted

- You feel "stuck"

- Life doesn't feel joyful

- You cling to the idea of being right

- You live within the good/bad right/wrong paradigm

- You find yourself in unfulfilling or toxic relationships

- You find connecting with other people difficult

- You feel like something is missing

- Your beliefs are keeping you caged

- The false self/ego = A reactionary life.

- The Infinite Self = A life of choice.

Don't fall into the habit of thinking there is something wrong with you or there is a problem. The ego loves that. Just be present with it and observe what is from your observer perspective.

To be clear, ego work is not something that comes quickly. Ego work is a shift in consciousness, a shift in identity that happens over time. For me, the ego first kicked and screamed and was angry, pissy, and vicious. Then it softened and became almost shy and apologetic, then it became playful and childlike, until eventually all identity was removed. I then found myself as the aware presence, residing in a fun, quirky, and beautiful physical persona.

Returning the Ego Back to Faculty

So the first order of business is to wake up from your nap and hop back in the driver's seat. Wipe the sleep out of your eyes, put on your seat belt, and get excited and ready for the wild ride called partnering with the mind and mastering physicality. Approaching it in this way lightens the mood and makes working with the mind adventurous and fun instead of horrific.

You are learning to facilitate the mind and ego so it does what it is meant to do: get more information. NOT repeat old outdated and untrue information. Most people listen to thoughts like they are real and listen to the lies instead of discerning and directing.

LAURI-ISM: The ego can be trained in 40 days with diligent awareness and discernment.

It took me over a year and I still get tempted to identify with the information received at times and get hooked. Identity and no-identity is sticky business! Don't worry about how long it will take you. Just put on your seat belt and do your best to enjoy the ride. The more you can laugh with and love the ego, the sooner it loses identity and becomes a willing partner. Here is an exercise my clients find helpful in interrupting ego activity.

The Ego Interrupt

The following can help you discern between true self and ego activity:

Ego Activity	True Self /Aware Discerner
Fear, Dread	Unconditional Love, Safety
Uncertainty, Anxiety	Certainty, Inner Knowing, Intuition
Anger, Frustration, Stress	
Difficulty	Calm
Guilt and Shame	Ease
Judgment, Lack	Peace
Self-Doubt, Worry	Acceptance, Allowance, Fullness
Apathy, Resignation, Cynicism	No Identity/Isness
	Freedom
Hopelessness	Joy
Sadness, Loneliness	Empty, Yet Full
I Have to/Need to, Should/ Shouldn't	Infinite Possibilities
	I Choose
Right/Wrong, Good/Bad	In Flow
The Need to Control	Human Being, Is-ness, Inspired Action
Human Doing Activity	
Energy in the Headspace, Mental Activity	Energy in the Heart Space, Calm
Closed, Resistance, Contraction	Open, Allowance, Expansion
	Wisdom
Unreasonable	Contentment, Complete
Lack, Scarcity, More, More, More	Lives in the Present Moment
	Knows You are Safe
Lives in the Past and Future	Absence of All Story, Meaning and Identity
Wants to Protect	
Stories and Meaning Given to Create Identity	

If you experience anything in the left hand column you know

you are in ego. The activities in the right column represent your true self as the aware presence. When you experience ego activity, get emotionally triggered, or get caught up in an ego loop where you think about the same thing over and over again, like a dog chewing on a bone, you've lost your position as the aware discerner.

When you get hooked by the ego, use this process to interrupt ego activity and return to your position as the aware discerner.

The Ego Interrupt: STOP! Cultivate awareness. Take a slow, deep, relaxing breath, and let go of the information brought to you by the ego. Swipe left, flick it off your shoulder, breathe it out, drop your shoulders, whatever you need to do to let that information go and move on with your day.

If you get hooked or triggered by the information the ego brings you or thrashes you with, INCREASE YOUR AWARENESS of what's happening (you're caught up in ego activity) Turn up the dial on awareness so that you are fully present in the room. Notice the sounds in the room, the fan, the creaking walls etc. SHIFT your attention from your headspace to your body by feeling your feet, your legs, your butt, your crotch. See if you can feel the beat of your heart. This will pull you out of the headspace where the ego lives into your body and the aware presence that is you. Cultivating awareness raises your level of consciousness where you rise above ego activity and can watch the information come and go without getting hooked by it. The less attention you give the ego, the easier it is to let go of the information it brings you and enjoy your day. The more you struggle with it the more discomfort you will experience.

It's Not Work: It's awareness and letting go. When you send the ego unconditional love and acceptance, it melts. It truly is well intentioned and wants to keep you safe. Don't resist the ego. Put your hand on your heart and thank it sincerely while you swipe left on the information it brings you repeatedly. This trains the ego to stop bringing you old information repetitively.

Optional Challenge: Once you have broken the loop and are in a space of calm, think of something you love. Something easy like puppies, food, friends, family, etc. If you feel resistance to feeling good see if you can push beyond it and allow yourself to embrace well-being. You could also do a gratitude rant and go on a litany of all the things you are thankful for. GET FAMILIAR WITH FEELING GOOD and opening your heart.

You are the Creator of Your Life: You create with your thoughts, and you do have the power to choose these. It takes awareness to break the pattern of unconscious creating and become the conscious creator of your life. Often we are entrained to ego activities unconsciously and it can be frustrating when we discover this. Now that you are aware and back in the seat as the discerner, you get to choose how you feel at all times.

LAURI-ISM: You are the creator of your life. Does what you are creating make you happy to lay your head on the pillow at night? If not, then it's up to you to choose something different. Only you can do it.

Tips

Thank the Ego: Thank the ego for wanting to keep you safe, and swipe left on information that doesn't serve you. Eventually you will be working as a team so the more you treat your ego like a faculty of the mind the easier it will be.

Cultivate Awareness: Observing the ego is the quickest way to dissolve it and return it to the faculty it originated as. All illusion disappears when exposed to pure consciousness. No false identity can withstand it, not one. No matter what the ego argues for or the emotions that arise as a result, when you become aware of the egoic thought, belief, or behavior pattern you detach from it and it loses its power. The more conscious you can be when these patterns arise, the more they dissolve. I mentioned the importance of cultivating awareness, didn't I?

Be Present: Another way to deal with the ego is to be in the present moment. The ego lives in the past and the future. The ego attaches to things in the future that will enhance its identity. It will also attach to things in the past that give it identity. It is never satisfied. But when you are fully in the present moment, it can't create meaning or be in story.

Direct the Mind: The mind is too limited to understand that the information it brings you is not helpful. It needs training and direction. Always swipe left on what doesn't serve you and ask it to retrieve new and better information, not bring you the same old repetitive information. You have access to every piece of information on earth and in the great universe. All you have to do is direct your mind and receive it. Ask and it is given!

Rest in No Thought: A side effect of ego work is a quiet mind, which is deeply relaxing and enjoyable. Get comfortable resting in the space between thoughts. Explore it. There is great peace and contentment here for you.

Let Go of Your Identity: Let go of your identity as a mother, a father, a healer, a worker, a husband, or wife. Let go of your identity as successful, not successful, rich, or poor. Let go of any identity that limits you or puts you in a box. Especially the identity as a spiritual or enlightened being. This almost always brings up the question, "Well then, who am I?" You are conscious awareness or attention. You are the awareness that navigates emotions without fear of losing your identity because you have none.

Remove All Identity from the Ego: When we give the ego identity we give it power. Removing all identity from the ego, even the so-called positive identities, and recognizing it for what it truly is—a faculty that brings you information—can help return it to its rightful and honored role as a bringer of information.

Don't Take Dismantling the Ego Too Seriously: You have to approach this process with a sense of humor. When you step back into your role as discerner, the information the mind brings you in the form of thoughts, ideas, and beliefs can be quite entertaining. You will find yourself laughing hilariously at the ridiculous things you let slip by before. Don't berate yourself, just keep swiping left, and laughing.

Get Familiar with Your True Self: Spend time sitting with yourself and being the aware presence that is you. Be curious about this thing called consciousness. What is this thing called the essence of you that lies beyond thoughts, beliefs, ideas, and emotions? Become aware of every moment of every day what is going on in both your inner and outer worlds.

Choose: Instead of reacting to the world around you, choose the actions you take. Taking back your seat as the chooser puts you in the role of active creator of your life. You are no longer unconsciously reacting to events and the world around you, but consciously choosing what to do based on your preferences. You choose based on what you prefer instead of what other people think you should choose. This is the return to authenticity.

Be Aware of the Ego: Identify your ego and observe how it drives your reactions. Until this point in your life, you've been mostly unaware of your ego. When you're unconscious (for most people this is 95% of the time) your ego is running the show. Only through being consciously aware of your ego and observing the ego can you dismantle it. You realize that is simply a reactionary pattern, not who you are. This can bring a sense of deep peace. The ego does not like to be observed, so observing it is very uncomfortable. Mostly because you think the behaviors and maneuvers of the ego is who you are. Think of the ego as autopilot that you have let take over while you were on vacation. Now that you are back, the house is a mess from all the parties, and it's time to clean up by cultivating awareness, removing identity, and swiping left.

What to Expect: It can be difficult in the beginning to break a pattern. It's frustrating, and takes effort to move through discomfort. Be compassionate with yourself and patient with your mind as you go through this process. It does get easier over time. It is not work; it's awareness, compassion, acceptance, and letting go. In the beginning you may notice an egoic thought or behavioral pattern after you have acted it out and experienced an emotional trigger. Continue to cultivate awareness and the next time it arises you will notice yourself in the middle of it, and then later you may catch it before it happens. The voice of the ego will also get finer and finer as you retrain it and it returns to the faculty it originated as.

MEDITATION: Ego Observation 1

This is one of my favorite things to do when I want to know exactly where I am with my character and whether I have attached to anything.

1. Find a quiet place with no distraction where you can sit in silence and in stillness for 30 minutes.
2. On a pad of paper, create two columns. Label one Thoughts and the other Emotions.
3. Wait for the ego to present itself in the form of a thought. This can be in the form of a complaint, an excuse, or a reason to get up and not do the exercise. Thoughts trigger emotions so if you experience an emotion you will be able to witness how thoughts trigger emotions.
4. Every time the ego presents itself in the form of a thought that triggers an emotion, write down the thought or emotion in the appropriate column. For example, the thought, This is ridiculous, may arise, triggering the emotion of frustration. Put ridiculous in the thought column and frustration in the emotion column. Fear, judgment, worry, blame, victim, guilt, shame, anger, self-flatulation, monkey mind, uncertainty, etc. are things you may write

down that describe the emotion you experience. When you experience the same thought or emotion over and over again, just put a checkmark next to the thought or emotion.

5. If any discomfort arises, increase your awareness and remember, you are the observer. If you get hooked or triggered and end up down the rabbit hole experiencing an intense emotion, focus on your breathing, cultivate awareness, and use the 5-Step Dissipater. It will return you to the observer's seat where you will rise above it. It is important to know the emotion will always dissipate.

6. After 30 minutes, look at what's on paper. This exercise will give you a bird's eye view of the ego and how it uses thoughts and emotions to manipulate you.

7. Now on another piece of paper write down two columns, one for Thoughts and one for Emotions. In each column write down the opposite of what you observed. For instance, if judgment was in one column you would write down acceptance. If you experienced fear, you would write down love. If I can't was a thought, you would write I can. When you are done, you are witnessing an alternative possible reality for the character you call you. Notice how this exercise takes your body through a wide range of vibrational frequencies and emotional experiences.

Congratulations! You just witnessed the ego and how this faculty of the mind brings you information. Practice is key with this new skill. The repetition will dissolve old pathways in the brain and create new pathways that allow observation and discernment to come more easily with time. It can be very uncomfortable to experience yourself as the observer at first. You might feel sensations in your body or racing thoughts telling you not to practice the exercise. All of this is totally normal, fear-based resistance from the ego. Seeing your ego is the first step in the dismantling process.

Note: Both pages of paper represent possible characters that you could assume. Don't get caught up in one identity or another. Both are false identities. Both are possible ways you could navigate through life. This exercise is to show you that you create the character that you call you, and if you are going to create a character to navigate this physical world, why not create a good one and wear it loosely?

What to Expect with Ego Observation: In the beginning you may notice a conditioned behavior, such as beating yourself up, and it may be an intense experience. Then, as your awareness increases, you catch yourself in the middle of the activity. Then, as you improve, you can catch it before it happens and the intensity will decrease. It's like the voice of the ego slowly fades away and gets fainter, leaving you and the mind to work in partnership. You may have major breakthroughs during this observation stage.

The Ego and Time

Another way to work with the ego is to be in the present moment. The ego lives in the past and in the future. The ego attaches to things in the future that will enhance its identity. It will also attach to things in the past that give it identity. It is never satisfied. But when you can be fully in the present moment. It can't survive. When you become aware of the inner self as presence, as consciousness, and disidentify from the ego, it quiets.

How can you be in the present moment? When you have a memory of the past, when are you remembering it? Now. The past is a now-moment that has already gone by. When you think about what might happen in the future, when are you thinking of it? Now. When that future thing happens, when does it happen? Now. So all we have is now. The ego is always attached to the past or the future, so the way out is to exist in the now. There's nothing wrong with memories; it is the identification with them that can be problematic and limiting.

You escape the ego by becoming aware of the ego and practice being in the present moment as much as possible. Ego and awareness are incompatible.

MEDITATION: Ego Observation 2

This is another fun exercise you can do to find out how much time your mind spends in the past, the present, or future.

1. Find a quiet place with no distraction where you can sit in silence and in stillness for 10 minutes.
2. The ego loves to time travel or judge what is happening. On a pad of paper draw three columns. Label one column past hurts or grievances. Label one column present dissatisfactions. Label the third column future fantasies. Each time the ego time

travels or judges your present situation, put a check mark in the appropriate column. This will tell you where you spend most of your time. The more you do this, the more you will experience moments of "no thought" where you escape time and are fully present in the now and the number of checks in the columns will decrease. Could have, should have, would have are past tense and the need to, have to, and should do are future tense phrases the ego loves.

3.   In those moments of no thought, be curious. What is it like to be in silent stillness at that point before thought?

The Triggered Ego

A trigger is an emotional response not equal to or way out of proportion to an event. A trigger tells you that the ego has been activated.

The ego is a master storyteller. It has thousands and thousands of emotional events and experiences logged that you can't consciously remember. These stories are supposed to serve to protect you from a future event, but they really don't. Instead, they always keep you tied to your past experiences and make the present situation worse.

The next time you are triggered, pay attention to the experience. You will know you are triggered when you have a faster heartbeat, you feel like yelling/shutting down, or have a feeling you might "lose" it.

Here is a simple worksheet that can help you work through a trigger:

I felt the emotion _____
when _____
The event of _____
means _____ .

Here is an example:
I felt the emotion anger when my partner left the dishes in the sink.

The event of leaving the dishes in the sink means that I am not worthy of consideration.

The objective reality was that dishes were left in the sink. This caused the emotion anger because of an underlying belief that "I am not worthy of consideration."

Here, the mind reacted to the situation and a thought arose that triggered an emotional response (based on a past framework of unworthiness). This was painful, and since you've never learned to process emotion, the ego projected it outwards and responded by calling your partner a slob. Your ego prefers to dump emotions on others, rather than feel a painful emotion within yourself.

The best way to deal with a trigger is to just ride it out until the chemicals released by the event die down. Don't react, don't project, don't blame or lose your shit. Allow yourself to feel your emotions and let them move through you.

Practice the 5-Step Dissipater. It's the trigger killer.

Then when the storm of the emotion has moved through and out of you, you can receive the gift and decipher what that trigger is trying to tell you about your life and belief systems.

In this situation you may learn that you have allowed yourself to get stuck in a pattern of doing other people's dishes and are doing something you don't want to do and blaming them while taking on feelings of unworthiness. Once you see your situation from a new perspective you can then choose how you want to respond instead of a knee jerk reaction.

Go Slowly and Reassure the Ego it Doesn't Die

When you use the strategies, meditations and suggestions in this book, be gentle and go slow. Peel away identity a little bit at a time gradually. To make the ego feel safe, reassure it that it does not die, it transforms and you work as a team. It has the ability to access new and exciting information throughout the universe instead of repeating old information. This can be an exciting concept to help its transition.

INTEGRATION: Practice the ego interrupt and do the meditations suggested in this chapter before moving on. It is normal to have mystical experiences and experience yourself in ways you never imagined. Yes. What you experience is real. More real than the illusions you are dismantling.

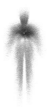

CHAPTER 12:

THE EGO, PART THREE

Quick Recap: In order to transmute the ego it must be stable. We talked about the three types of ego, and the many activities of the ego to help you identify when you are in ego or not. We talked about how to remove identity from the ego gradually and in a way that makes it feel safe, thus returning it back to the faculty it originated as. You learned a valuable strategy called The Ego Interrupt, as well as other exercises and tips on how to handle the ego effectively. You were given two meditations designed to observe the ego and experience how the ego cannot exist in the now. You discovered that triggers tell you when your ego has been activated and how the 5- Step Dissipater is the trigger killer.

Do you feel integrated with this? Right on! Let's keep going.

Appreciating the Ego

Appreciation helps the transition from an unhealthy ego to a healthy ego, where it can then be removed of identity leaving you and the mind to work as an integrated team. When you wrap your arms around the ego with unconditional love and acceptance, no matter how dark the thought, belief, emotion, or behavior, it quickly softens.

Here's an example of what ego appreciation might look like in our example of dishes in the sink: Thank you, ego, for bringing me this information in the form of this trigger and trying to protect me. I see the situation from my place as the discerner. All is well. I've got this. There are dishes in the sink. It doesn't mean anything about who I am or who this other person is. Can you bring me a new perspective on how to handle this, please?

Once you have calmed down, you, as the observer, get to choose your response. This is a much higher quality response because it is based on personal choice, not a knee jerk reaction.

You get to choose: "Do I do the dishes or leave them for the person who left them? What other possible choices are available to me?"

Asking the question, "How can I step out of this pattern?" can also be helpful.

When I owned the wellness center many of my employees left unclean dishes in the sink. After many requests that went unheeded and many triggered emotions, I made the new rule that any dishes in the sink would be thrown out. This went for other personal items that cluttered community spaces. Soon enough there were no dishes and people had to bring their own and wash their own or they would be thrown out. This worked like a charm. Soon everyone was responsible for their own dishes.

The ego doesn't bring you information about anyone else. It is ALWAYS about you. While it may want to project, blame, or judge, what it is telling you about yourself is that you are in a pattern of projecting, blaming, or judging, or doing something you don't want to do. When you see what is going on within you from your place as the discerner, you separate from the pattern knowing it is not you but a pattern that was created when you fell asleep in the back seat. Now instead of reacting unconsciously, you choose your response or decide not to respond at all.

Again, it is worth repeating: when you become aware of the thought, belief, or behavior pattern it loses its power. The more conscious you can be when these patterns arise, the more they can be dismantled and let go. The ego then becomes a way for you to know where you are with yourself.

LAURI-ISM: The ego is nothing more than an energy-giving opportunity.

Benefits of Ego Work

- Ego work transitions you from a life of reaction to personal choice and responsibility.

- Because your ego is no longer in the driver's seat you become more and more familiar with your true self. Life gets easier, simpler, and synchronicities become more apparent that enrich your life.

- Confidence and self-love result from being in the driver's seat.

- You transition from low vibe emotions to high vibe emotions. You feel good.

- You experience more moments of stillness, a quiet mind, peace, and a constant joyful inner beingness.

- Problems and attachments fall away.

- Life gets simpler and easier.

- Most importantly, the ego transitions from an unruly identity to a useful faculty called the mind.

Releasing Judgments

Personality constructs often arise in relation to the roles we have chosen to play in life. Husband, wife, victim, perpetrator, significant, insignificant, successful, rich, poor, and so on.

The ego loves to judge and identify as bad. If you've done something in your life that you are not proud of, guilt and shame may be constant companions. I have worked with many people who at one time in their life perpetrated some offense and it haunts them unnecessarily. We have all played both sides of the perpetrator/victim card. And we have all gained wisdom from both experiences that give rise to preference and clarity. Letting go of the construct of good/bad, right/wrong enables us to see the world from a higher perspective. A cause and effect perspective where the effect results from the vibrational alignment with our intentions of what we want to cause.

Storytime: Once upon a time there was a God up in heaven that gave all of its beautiful souls freedom to experience anything they wanted just for the experience of it. He created an amusement park with all kinds of rides for them to choose from. No good or bad or right or wrong, just experience for the sake of experience. Some souls took the Ferris wheel, some went through the haunted house. Some did both. All gained wisdom and insights into what they liked and disliked. Sometimes the souls did crazy things and God just looked at them like beloved children and shook his head and laughed. One day there were two souls hanging out in heaven. One soul says to the other soul, "Hey, let's forget who we are and incarnate into physical form and play cops and robbers. I'll be the good guy and you will be the bad guy." The other soul agrees and they incarnate, have the experience, and when it's all over they come sliding back into heaven, remember who they really are and start laughing at the experience and how they took it all so seriously. They gained much clarity on what they liked and disliked. They gained wisdom.

Imagine being completely unlimited, then extremely limited, only to experience yourself as unlimited again in a whole new way. It brings new meaning to the words, "Who am I?"

How fun is this? What wisdom and contrast would you gain about yourself by forgetting yourself and then remembering?

What clarity would you gain regarding what you like and don't like?

LAURI-ISM: Wisdom is the knowing all is of the same resource, using the same material, having unique experiences creating unique value, shaping and shifting all valued meanings over time.

This story can be helpful when we look at our life and remember things we have done that we may not be proud of. For instance, I had a client once who cheated on his wife and it haunted him day after day after day. I told him the story of cops and robbers and that there was no good or bad, only wisdom gained. Then

I asked him, "What wisdom have you gained?" He immediately smiled and said, "Not to ever do that again!" The relief from judgment and shame was palpable. His shoulders dropped and I could tell he was instantly freed from any identity he had projected onto himself as bad.

REFLECTIVE MOMENT: What wisdom have you gained from your life experiences?

I have a sister, who for many years, was with a man who beat her. He would get angry, drag her across the floor by her foot, hit her in the face, and slam her fingers in the door. One day I flew into town to help her get away from this person. She had left him many times but always went back. Perhaps this time was different. So my other sister and I got her set up in an apartment, filled her fridge with food, and helped her with her budget so she could be self-sufficient. Later I discovered that she went back to him and was hiding it from the rest of the family. I was so frustrated. I couldn't believe she would go back after all he had put her through. One day I was on a call with Lauri and this is what she said:

LAURI-ISM: You have no idea what the soul contract may be between those two. She could have agreed to be a steadfast companion for him while he worked out his distortions.

This was a much higher perspective that made sense to me and helped me look at the situation differently. It gave me compassion for him and a greater appreciation for her. Years later, he got cancer and died quite suddenly. My sister was extremely angry that he had died so soon after finally getting his anger under control. According to her, he had finally worked out his distortions.

My point with these two stories is that when we remove the judgments of good and bad and right and wrong, we free ourselves from judgment, and the guilt and shame that goes with it. Experience becomes wisdom gained. In fact true wisdom can only be gained from experience.

Where have you played the victim in your life?

What wisdom have you gained? What strength, clarity, or quality did you receive as a gift from that experience?

Where have you played the perpetrator in your life?

What wisdom have you gained? What strength, clarity, or quality did you receive as a gift from that experience?

How does looking at life from the perspective of there is no good or bad change things?

When you recognize the story you have told about yourself or the role you have chosen to play, whether consciously or unconsciously, and are ready to tell a new story or assume a new role, you must cultivate awareness regularly to interrupt that old story. Awareness dissolves all illusions.

When you look at life from this perspective instead of good or bad, right or wrong, you see there is only experience and wisdom gained. No one is bad because they cut me off in traffic. No one is wrong because they have millions of dollars in their bank account. No one is bad because they are homeless, addicted to drugs, in a relationship that causes suffering, or living the life of their dreams. In a sense, we are all living the life of our dreams. The question is, "Are we living it consciously, or is our life being directed by a false identity called the ego because we fell asleep in the back seat?"

Ego and Emotions

Often when emotion arises it is because of something that happened in the past that we have given meaning to and we are bringing that experience into our now-moment. For instance, you had a date in the past that didn't go well. He was good looking and very nice, but he didn't want to see you again and you felt rejected. So, anytime you have a date now a fear pops up that "Oh no, I'm going to get rejected."

To get beyond this, you address all emotions without a story. Addressing emotions without a story can bypass ego activity and false identity. This magically addresses the past, too. For example, the fear arises that "I'm going to get rejected." You notice this emotional information brought to you by the ego in the form of fear. You notice it is designed to keep you safe, thank it, accept that it is there, and observe it as it fades into the background. Swipe left.

There is no such thing as rejection, only preference and

experience that you and others get to choose. There is no meaning if this person chooses not to see you again, or if you choose not to see them. You felt the fear, then immediately stripped it of all meaning.

Byron Katie's The Work is fabulous at stripping meaning from emotions. You can ask the questions, "Is this true, I'm going to get rejected? Can I absolutely know this is true?" No. "How do I feel when I have that thought?" Usually not so good. "Who would I be without this thought, I'm going to get rejected?" I would be going on a date. Period. You may even transform the meaning and add as the turnaround, "I'm not going to get rejected," or "What a great opportunity to meet someone new regardless of what happens." Again, if you are going to create a story, why not create a good one?

When you energetically explore and work with limiting belief structures, you will notice they are all composed of low frequency emotions, such as fear, doubt, anxiety, worry, frustration, jealousy, apathy, feelings of inadequacy, etc. Facing them with an elevated awareness enables you to see the structure from a new perspective. Gratitude naturally arises as you witness the transformation of meaning. Emotions literally transform from something you thought was bad or unwanted to something that is bringing you valuable information about yourself and where you are. This is alchemy. It's what people mean when they say, "face the shadow." You must face the low frequency emotions to receive the information they bring to process that information and transcend it. You are then open to experience higher frequency emotions, such as contentment, optimism, positive expectation, gratitude, and love. The shadow or darkness is the light. It's just lower on the vibrational scale.

The Dalai Lama once said, "Pain is inevitable. Suffering is optional." This is true and a really good example of the role the ego plays in our suffering. For instance, the inevitability of pain in our life arises when someone dies or leaves the relationship or we have an illness. The experience may be painful. It's only when the ego attaches to the situation, identifies with it and gives meaning to it such as, "Poor me. I am all alone now. It must be about me. I must not be worthy," that the suffering begins.

When you practice the 5-Step Dissipater to face your emotions and do The Work on emotions to strip them of meaning it helps you address emotions without a story and holds you firmly in the seat of the discerner and chooser of your reality.

The transformation of the ego is really only a matter of outgrowing a personality or false self.

Many people know there is more to them than meets the eye, yet never allow themselves to experience it as truth. Yet we know it to be true. In our heart of hearts we know we have a little slice of God within us.

The Ego and Fear

You may question as you step into this space of no identity, what will happen to me? How will I survive, how will I make money? This is the voice of the ego in fear and conjecture about the future. This is supposition and is not knowing. Fear and the ego find conjecture highly useful. When you align to fear you align to the possibility of what you'd rather not experience. The ego loves fear as a way to keep you safe. If you never take a risk, you will never fail.

Fear is a figment of your imagination. The action of fear is and always has been to create more fear. Recall that thoughts trigger emotions and emotions trigger more thoughts in a feedback loop. These are low vibrational thoughts and emotions that have simply been entrained in you since your youth in response to your parents and the world around you. When you claim who you are as divine and choose to be in alignment with the higher frequencies of love there is no fear because you have lifted beyond your lower vibratory form. Life beyond fear is very attainable and a life in expression as the divine is your birthright.

To transmute fear when it arises, you simply acknowledge it. "Oh fear is arising." Non-attachment. The 5-Step Dissipater transmutes fear to truth very effectively because you detach from fear and become the witnesser of fear.

Practicing non-attachment is the answer. When people avoid fear, it's like avoiding love. But when you avoid fear and then don't avoid love you are repressing one and experiencing the other, and there is judgment. Fear is bad and love is good. This is the attachment to an idea of something being good or bad. When you experience your emotions you want to experience them ALL and receive the gift of what they are trying to tell you.

I have heard it said that fear is the same thing as excitement. It is the same emotion with two different stories attached to it. Makes sense, doesn't it?

When you experience love, experience it fully. Love is arising. Experience it without meaning or attachment. If you receive love it doesn't mean anything. It doesn't mean you're a good person or did something right. Experience love without attachment. For instance, if I empty out the garbage I'll get love. (Condition, meaning, attachment, and expectation.) We set up the expectation that in the future if I do this, I will get love. And we get attached to an outcome that we will get love, but that's not love, that's agenda. So we've taken an experience that is so beautiful and so magical that arises within us spontaneously and we use it to manipulate.

We do the same thing with fear. When you experience fear, experience it fully. Fear is arising. Experience it without meaning or attachment. If you experience fear it doesn't mean anything, it doesn't mean you should or shouldn't do something or you are a fearful person. No, fear is just arising. Experience fear without attachment of a story. For instance, if I don't behave in a certain way I'll get rejected. (Condition, meaning, attachment, and expectation.)

We also attach to fear because we think it helps us navigate so love isn't withdrawn and we can stay safe. That's also an agenda and manipulation. It is an agenda at the cost of authenticity and expression. Fear is almost always telling us where we have sacrificed ourselves, given away ourselves, are not expressing ourselves, or not experiencing what we really desire to experience.

REFLECTIVE MOMENT: How has fear limited your expression, authenticity, or ability to experience life?

Identity Crisis and Transition of Identity

The integration process you are undertaking is the release of the false self/ego structure and allowance of your true self to be known. This is a wonderful and joyful process that involves acclimating to the higher frequencies as you paradoxically know yourself as that which can never be known.

It can also lead to an identity crisis where everything you thought you were collapses so your true self can come through. I work with many people who are at this place, and while it is uncomfortable, it is a moment worthy of congratulations. The feeling of being lost, yet found, not knowing who they are, yet sensing something indescribable within. Identity crisis is a normal experience when the ego returns to the faculty of the mind, and the uncertainty of who you are arises. This opens a space for self-discovery and integration of true self.

You must die to the false self for the true self to be known. This is what some call enlightenment.

I was visiting Mt. Shasta to hike recently and a gal that I met invited me to lunch with her and her friends. At lunch one of the girls asked, "What was your experience of awakening like?" And as each of us shared it gave us all reassurance that we weren't going crazy. We were just waking up.

There are many people in the world who feel alone and scared to share their experiences for fear others will think they are crazy. People are having transcendent meditation experiences and extraordinary insights and knowings. Channeling is more common than ever and the awakened state will soon be described as the new normal. So let this text reassure you. If you are having an identity crisis, it is probably a very good thing! Let it fall apart. Cultivate awareness and come home to your true self.

Once you release identity, all identity, even your identity as a spiritual person, you can align more and more to who and what you really are. Sure, you'll flop back and forth for a while. That is completely expected. When you find yourself striving to be pious or good, watch out. That's also the ego wanting to attach to an identity as spiritual, significant, or better than others.

LAURI-ISM: So often we think we need to be pious, holy, or act a certain way to awaken. Consider Jesus. He wasn't pious. He drank wine, had sex, laughed, and celebrated life. He was a walking example of all the possibilities before you.

Stop judging what you do and take off the character you have created that is limited. You are not limited by anyone or anything but yourself.

Ego Integration

Many of my clients say that they feel like they have a split personality or that there are two of them residing in a physical body because the voice of the ego is so strong and dominant. Those that engage with this voice and indulge in the information being brought to them have the hardest time.

They will bargain, argue with it, and allow themselves to be bombarded with all kinds of false information. So let's get really clear on this. ANY TIME you talk to yourself it is the voice of a false identity seeking to maintain its existence. The more you cultivate awareness of the voice and pay it no mind the quicker it will dissolve.

In the beginning it is very helpful to reassure the ego, to show it compassion because it has taken on a life of its own, an energetic entity you thought was you. As you work with the ego and gently strip it of identity and approach it like a faculty of the mind the sooner it will transform. This means not giving it too much attention and redirecting it over and over again in a detached way.

Dealing with the ego for me went in phases. At first I struggled with it, fought it, and treated it like an evil part of me I wanted to kill with a hatchet. Once I realized this didn't work I began talking with and reasoning with it. Most of the time I lost because it was so skilled at triggering emotional responses that reinforced old habits and patterns to which I had become addicted. The ego is very clever. Then I began to love the ego and gently said, "Nope. I love you, but that's not what we are doing." I accepted it was there and began to navigate it like an unruly child that just needed parenting. This was helpful because when I loved the ego and parented it like a child, it stopped fighting me and transitioned from something that was constantly thrashing me and beating me up to an apologetic entity that didn't know any better. Then I noticed that once it felt loved and accepted it actually became playful.

I realized at this point that I was in a relationship with myself—my true self engaging with the entity or persona called Dani that had taken on a life of its own. I saw differently the personality structure I had created. I saw the scared little girl, the angry teenager, the hurt young woman who felt she had to conform. I saw how that wasn't my true self but what I had created based on how I perceived events and situations throughout my life. The persona called Dani was actually beautiful. I had tried to rocket launch the Dani. My own creation of me. I had judged it, rejected it, and wanted it to be different than it was. I had denied Dani.

Now Lauri had told me many times that I needed a persona while navigating the physical realm, but someone can tell you something a hundred times until all of a sudden it lands within you as a knowing. This is what happened. At that point I started observing Dani. I saw how the persona I had created while I slept was actually pretty cool. Sure, she had insecurities. In fact, she was quite shy, a bit scared, and uncertain what was happening. The more I watched her without judgment, the more I noticed her quirkiness. She liked to sing in the kitchen, make up strange songs and dance like a weirdo. She liked hot baths, walks in nature, lying in the sunshine, and reading books. She was a voracious learner. And she loved to write. She also liked to drink and smoke and had a tendency to be a know-it-all. She went back and forth between I am not worthy and I've totally got this.

So I made friends with this entity called Dani. I saw that ego was Dani, the persona I had created while I slept. I laughed with her and at her. I shook my head like God must shake his head at the silliness of humanity, and we developed trust. I did mirror work and every time I looked into my own eyes I learned something new. I let the anger come; I let the tears fall as I held the creation called Dani.

I started to wear her loosely. The more I observed her the closer we got until one day we started to meld. Her voice slowly receded into the background and the two voices became one. I started to reside in being, stillness, peace, and knowing. Again, ANYTIME you talk to yourself it is the voice of a false identity seeking to maintain its existence. But that doesn't mean the false identity is bad. No. Quite on the contrary. It is the delicate tender and beautiful creation called you that formed while you slept.

The persona called Dani that I wear loosely is a wonderful creation that enables me to experience physicality and interact with others. I get to touch, taste, kiss, and experience things in this realm that are not available to me in non physical. I get to experience you as a unique expression, and you get to experience me. We get to experience Oneness as individual expressions. It's another paradox and it's beautiful beyond words.

LAURI-ISM: If you were floating around in the cosmos as one infinite being, wouldn't you want to separate yourself so that you had others to share with?

I know that what resides within me lies within all beings, all things. Now, my physical form is slow to adapt, but it is learning. I am still working out the kinks, the energetic emotional hairballs, the belief structures of the past, and I am learning to use my mind as the faculty it is to bring me new and exciting information. My intuitive abilities have shot through the roof and I am excited to see what else this physical body can do.

The voice in my head continues to get fainter and fainter and I really have to focus to catch the little nuances of the false identities as they fade away. The craziest thing I face now is freedom of choice. I sometimes still get paralyzed and uncertain as to what I want to create, what I want to experience, what I want to call forth as a free, sovereign, infinite being. I still like to sing in the kitchen, make up strange songs, and dance like a weirdo. I still like hot baths, walks in nature, lying in the sunshine, and reading books. I am not as much of a voracious learner now that I know all the answers are within me, and I am figuring out how to retrieve them. I still love to write. I also still enjoy bourbon and cigars, but I don't choose them as often. There is no need to or have to. Now, for me, it's all about choice, and to be honest, sometimes I feel so content that there doesn't seem to be anything to choose, but an unfolding to experience.

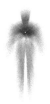

CHAPTER 13:

TRUE-SELF INTEGRATION

What I've discovered in my years on this planet is that who I am cannot be found in any of the roles I play. It cannot be found in a name, a label, or a concept. I am not the thoughts that go bouncing around in my head, and the emotions I experience as a result of those thoughts are nothing to be afraid of. In fact, they are quite the opposite. They are gifts that return me home to my true self.

Who I am is what's left after all the negative thoughts, limiting beliefs, and false identities are gone. From this place I found there was nothing left to do, nothing to become, and nothing to achieve. I experienced myself as nothing. Nothing. Absolutely nothing. This was startling at first and quite a shock. To be honest I was quite disappointed. Then, I laughed my ass off because my whole quest for enlightenment had ended in nothing! Imagine my reaction when I found enlightenment to be nothing! So I explored the nothing and found that within that nothing I still existed. And anything that came forth from this nothing was creation, including me. My mind wanted to add meaning to the nothing, but I resisted. I stayed in a place of no meaning. The more I explored the nothing, the more comfortable I got with it. I discovered that within the nothing was something...everything! The whole construct, the matrix, the planets, the galaxies, physical and non-physical, and the entire cosmos I found to be suspended in nothing. I was ecstatic to say the least, and for a brief moment I held the entire cosmos in the palm of my hand, turned around, and faced the infinite.

No, this was not under the influence of plant medicine. And yes, I am everything and nothing. So are you. And we are free to bring forth from the nothing anything we desire. It took me a while to acclimate to knowing myself as nothing and everything, I am still acclimating. At one point I found myself so fulfilled that even the desire to intend or create was gone. When you transition fully from identity to no identity the ego dissolves, the mind quiets, and you reside in stillness. Silence. No thinking mind that thrashes you, no need to, have to, shoulds or shouldn'ts. Just a soft lovely peace that resides in a great expansive beingness that is so utterly delicious you wish for nothing. So I hung out there for a while. I still hang out there today.

What has arisen for me from the nothing are new ways of

perceiving the world around me. I see who people are beyond any story they have about themselves. I see the world as a playground, and the goal, if there was one, is to have as much fun as possible. To experience as much love as this physical form can hold, and to open my heart to all that is, because it is. I no longer take life so seriously or think that highly of myself. I had spent so much of my life seeking and striving that when I finally found what I was looking for I burst out laughing. Today I carry with me a constant soft smile, a playful heart, and deep contentment. And surprisingly all those synchronicities that everyone talks about started to show up in my life...along with the stuff.

Do I still get hooked by false identity? Sure, we live in a realm of illusory separation and it's sticky here. But the more I anchor in the truth the less sticky it is. By truth I mean that I know who I am and I know what I am. I know who you are, too. We are absolutely nothing, relatively something, and the mystery in between. And it doesn't mean anything. It just is. And we are free to bring forth from the nothing anything we choose. We are the same, dear one. That which resides within us resides within all things. It is extraordinary, and it is ordinary.

Embodied Divinity

For the longest time in my meditations I would jet out of the physical and experience myself beyond space and time and physicality. It's just that good. But Lauri kept calling me back. Over and over again she reinforced that we know non-physical; that's where we came from. That the game we are here to win is to embody our divinity so that it can be expressed in the physical. So in my meditations I began to anchor my divinity into my body. I worked with it, played with it, laughed with it, and slowly integrated it. I am still integrating today. I don't believe there is a limit to the amount of joy, love, and ecstatic bliss this body can hold, and I'm having a ball with it! I also love resting in nothing. The void. The point before creation where I can let everything go and just be.

Enlightenment is when you let go of who you *think* you are in order to *know* what you are. It is when you know yourself as One, and yet function in the world as an individual. You are here for the experience of it, the experience of individuation. To share, to laugh, to love, to experience pain, sadness, suffering, and the whole gambit of life. All are worthy tickets to ride. We get trapped when we think we are the individual we came to play and get attached to what we create as who we are. This is why all the masters teach non attachment.

If you go into a deep meditation or do a plant medicine journey and experience your true self beyond your personality structure, there are no words. You cannot speak, let alone describe it. Yet when you come back into physical form you suddenly have words, the ability to share, express, and the contrast to know more about yourself in truth. I often experience wonder, amazement, grace, and enormous gratitude when I ponder how on earth the divine got all that into this physical body!

Understanding the nature of who you are when you are empty of all constructs is the first step in connecting with your true self. This, of course, is done with awareness.

I did mention the importance of cultivating awareness, didn't I?

Yes, we need a persona to function in this physical world as individuals. It is a paradox that we are One with all of creation, yet sovereign and individual. That we are everything and nothing. As the physical body slowly adapts to the higher vibrational frequencies, what it will be able to do is yet unknown. I scan the internet and see humans moving things with their minds, reading while blindfolded, and exploring remote viewing abilities. I witness healing through plant medicines on a regular basis and was thrilled to see a Youtube video of monks playing with their ability to walk on water. Humans are channeling in unprecedented numbers. Who knows, perhaps one day we will be able to project our consciousness across the galaxy and even appear there in form. Many ancient texts say this is possible.

The new human is extraordinary and ordinary. The matrix is changing!

Storytime: Imagine with me that all beings throughout the universe are like little kids in a sandbox, playing with toys and hitting each other over the head with their shovels, stealing each other's buckets, and building and destroying sand castles. A bunch of little kids not knowing who they are or what to do.

After taking turns hitting each other over the head and stomping on each other's castles, they realized that what they were doing wasn't working. They realized that everything they thought they were wasn't true. That all the distortions of fear, identity, lack, and limitation were false. They saw there are infinite resources and infinite things to create and experience. They saw that all creations were equal, unique, and beautiful and contributed to the diversity and richness of the whole. They experienced who they are beyond story and beyond identity and experienced themselves in Unity.

So they stood up, put down their shovels, and dropped their buckets, and wiping the sand off their faces, they began laughing. Laughing at the ridiculousness of it, hugging each other, and laughing because there was nothing to forgive. It didn't matter what happened in the past because they didn't know any better. They laughed at how many times they had hit others over the head with their shovels and how many times they had been hit over the head, and laughed some more. After the laughing stopped, they joined hands and hugged. They then asked the question, what now?

What now is undistorted creation.

Creation without fear, anxiety, or depression. Creation without self-doubt, guilt, or shame. Creation without judgment or comparison.

Can you imagine it?

Creation just for the sake of creating, not because you have to but because you choose to. Creation that vibrates in resonance with wisdom, unconditional love, and acceptance. Creation that celebrates individual expression, knowing full well we are all One. Because we are.

Welcome home!

Welcome to a new round of creation and the extraordinary, ordinary you!

ACKNOWLEDGMENTS

Much of the information in this book would not have made its way to me or to you without the help and guidance of my good friend and mentor Lauri Ivers. Thank you, Lauri, for being the crystal clear intuitive channel that you are, for your wisdom, friendship, and the Universal bitchslaps that served me so well.

Thanks to Jill L. Ferguson whose clarity, creativity, and eye for words on paper has contributed greatly to the energy in these pages. You never cease to amaze me, my friend!

Gratitude to Rick Schank for his beautiful cover design.

To the No Pants Girls Michelle Bingham Rhoads, Nayri Ishkhanian Geary, and Aydika James, I thank you for your reminders not to take things seriously and to NEVER forget to play.

Special thanks to my family: Mom for giving me the chutzpah to stand up to the world, Dad for teaching me to play, Kelly for her dedicated prayers, Stacy for hanging in there with me no matter how woo woo things got, James for bringing me laughter when I needed it the most, and Tori for teaching me the power of following your heart no matter what others think.

Immense Gratitude to Jonette Crowley, Mark, and Mike Putnam. You have contributed to my own awakening more than you will ever know!

Ingram Content Group UK Ltd.
Milton Keynes UK
UKHW021626060323
418095UK00014B/2016